MEDICAL MANAGEMENT OF

TYPE 2 DIABETES

SIXTH EDITION

MEDICAL MANAGEMENT OF

TYPE 2 DIABETES

SIXTH EDITION

Charles F. Burant, MD, PhD, Editor

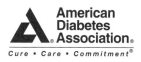

American Diabetes Association®
Cure • Care • Commitment®

Director, Book Publishing, Robert Anthony; *Associate Director, Professional Books*, Victor Van Beuren; *Managing Editor*, Abe Ogden; *Editor*, Gregory L. Guthrie; *Copyeditor*, Wendy M. Martin; *Production Manager*, Melissa Sprott; *Composition*, Circle Graphics, Inc.; *Cover Design*, Koncept, Inc.; *Printer*, Worzalla Publishing.

Printed in the United States of America
3 5 7 9 10 8 6 4

The suggestions and information contained in this publication are generally consistent with the *Clinical Practice Recommendations* and other policies of the American Diabetes Association, but they do not represent the policy or position of the Association or any of its boards or committees. Reasonable steps have been taken to ensure the accuracy of the information presented. However, the American Diabetes Association cannot ensure the safety or efficacy of any product or service described in this publication. Individuals are advised to consult a physician or other appropriate health care professional before undertaking any diet or exercise program or taking any medication referred to in this publication. Professionals must use and apply their own professional judgment, experience, and training and should not rely solely on the information contained in this publication before prescribing any diet, exercise, or medication. The American Diabetes Association—its officers, directors, employees, volunteers, and members—assumes no responsibility or liability for personal or other injury, loss, or damage that may result from the suggestions or information in this publication.

♾ The paper in this publication meets the requirements of the ANSI Standard Z39.48-1992 (permanence of paper).

ADA titles may be purchased for business or promotional use or for special sales. To purchase more than 50 copies of this book at a discount, or for custom editions of this book with your logo, contact the American Diabetes Association at the address below, at booksales@diabetes.org, or by calling 703-299-2046.

American Diabetes Association
1701 North Beauregard Street
Alexandria, Virginia 22311

Library of Congress Cataloging-in-Publication Data

Medical management of type 2 diabetes. — 6th ed.
    p. ; cm.
Rev. ed. of: Medical management of type 2 diabetes / Charles F. Burant, editor.
Includes bibliographical references and index.
ISBN 978-1-58040-310-8 (alk. paper)
1. Non-insulin-dependent diabetes. I. American Diabetes Association.
[DNLM: 1. Diabetes Mellitus, Type 2. WK 810 M48791 2008]

RC662.18.M43 2008
616.4'62—dc22

2008011391

Contents

Special Therapeutic Situations 87

Detection and Treatment of Chronic Complications 105

Behavior Change Strategies 139

Index 147

A Word About This Guide

Type 2 diabetes is now a worldwide epidemic. The increasing prevalence of obesity and sedentary lifestyles is a driving force in the dramatic increase of type 2 diabetes in our society. If these trends continue, one in three American children born in 2000 faces the probability of developing type 2 diabetes with the attendant risks of morbidity and early mortality. The care of individuals with diabetes will take an increasing portion of expenditures for health care, making this disease a problem for society as well as the individual. Reversing these trends will take a concerted effort in public education directed toward developing better lifestyle habits. The results of several studies have already shown that relatively small lifestyle changes to decrease caloric intake and increase exercise can slow or prevent the transition from impaired glucose tolerance to type 2 diabetes.

Although prevention of type 2 diabetes is a necessary key to addressing the epidemic, for the foreseeable future the practitioner will be caring for an increasing number of patients with diabetes. Since the last edition of this guide, there has been a significant increase in our knowledge of the pathogenesis of type 2 diabetes, its complications, and the options for treatment. Numerous studies have shown that lifestyle changes and pharmacological interventions make a significant impact on the well-being of the patient. Several cardiovascular intervention trials have demonstrated the importance, or even preeminence, of aggressive intervention with medications to control blood pressure and lipids, in addition to glucose, to prevent cardiovascular events in people with type 2 diabetes. It is also becoming clear that when diabetes needs to be treated with medications, multiple drugs can and should be used in combination to control hyperglycemia. The rapid introduction of additional medications when the first therapeutic options fail is of critical importance to control glucose in the short term and to prevent long-term complications. The recent introduction of medications that have unique mechanisms of action has made treatment of type 2 diabetes with oral agents easier and more effective. New insulin analogs and improved delivery devices that make insulin therapy safer and easier to use have increased patient acceptance and compliance. Using all available behavioral and therapeutic tools to improve the care of individuals with type 2 diabetes will likely save lives and decrease microvascular and macrovascular complications. Ultimately, this will improve the lives of those who have or are at risk for diabetes and decrease the cost to society.

This edition of *Medical Management of Type 2 Diabetes* has been updated to provide state-of-the-art information on these issues by a select group of experts. It also reflects the most recent *Clinical Practice Recommendations* from the American

Diabetes Association, including the diagnostic and classification criteria adopted by the Association in 2004. This book, along with other American Diabetes Association publications, including *Medical Management of Type 1 Diabetes, Therapy for Diabetes Mellitus and Related Disorders, Intensive Diabetes Management,* and *Medical Management of Pregnancy Complicated by Diabetes*, were designed to provide health care professionals with the comprehensive information needed to give the best possible medical care to patients with diabetes mellitus.

The American Diabetes Association believes that you will find this book as useful as its predecessors. We hope that it will encourage you to add other American Diabetes Association publications to your library, which can help you manage patients with diabetes more effectively.

CHARLES F. BURANT, MD, PhD
Editor

Contributors to the Sixth Edition

EDITOR

Charles F. Burant, MD, PhD
University of Michigan
Ann Arbor, Michigan

CONTRIBUTORS

Robert M. Anderson, EdD
University of Michigan
Ann Arbor, Michigan

Komen Benjamin, MPH, RD, LDN
University of North Carolina
Chapel Hill, North Carolina

John B. Buse, MD, PhD
University of North Carolina
Chapel Hill, North Carolina

Martha M. Funnell, MS, RN, CDE
University of Michigan
Ann Arbor, Michigan

Roma Gianchandani, MD
University of Michigan
Ann Arbor, Michigan

William Herman, MD, MPH
University of Michigan
Ann Arbor, Michigan

Robin B. Nwankwo, MPH, RD,
CDE
University of Michigan
Ann Arbor, Michigan

Rodica Pop-Busui, MD, PhD
University of Michigan
Ann Arbor, Michigan

Martin Stevens, MD
University of Birmingham
Birmingham, England

Jennifer Wyckoff, MD
University of Michigan
Ann Arbor, Michigan

Acknowledgments

The American Diabetes Association gratefully acknowledges the contributions of the following health care professionals and members of the Association's Professional Section to previous editions of this work:

Christine A. Beebe, MS, RD, CDE; Nathaniel G. Clark, MD, MS, RD; Mayer B. Davidson, MD; Harold E. Lebovitz, MD; David Nathan, MD; Philip Raskin, MD; Matthew C. Riddle, MD; Harold Rifkin, MD; Robert A. Rizza, MD; F. John Service, MD, PhD; Robert Sherwin, MD; and Bruce R. Zimmerman, MD.

The Association gratefully acknowledges the review by M. Sue Kirkman, MD.

Diagnosis and Classification

Highlights
Diagnosis and Classification

■ Diabetes is diagnosed on the basis of a random plasma glucose level ≥200 mg/dl (≥11.1 mmol/l) and symptoms of diabetes (polyuria, polydipsia, and unexplained weight loss), a fasting plasma glucose of ≥126 mg/dl (≥7.0 mmol/l), or a 2-h plasma glucose after a 75-g oral glucose tolerance test (OGTT) ≥200 mg/dl (≥11.1 mmol/l). The latter two tests should be confirmed on another day.

■ Diabetes is classified into two main types: type 1 diabetes, which has absolute insulin deficiency and a propensity to ketoacidosis, and type 2 diabetes, which is associated with relative insulin deficiency. The prevalence of type 2 diabetes increases with age and obesity. Type 2 diabetes is the most common form of diabetes, accounting for 90–95% of diabetes in Western societies.

■ Screening for diabetes using a fasting glucose should be performed every 3 years in individuals ≥45 years of age. More frequent and/or earlier screening with either a fasting glucose level or an OGTT should be considered in people with additional risk factors for diabetes.

■ Impaired fasting glucose (IFG) and impaired glucose tolerance (IGT) are used to describe individuals who have glucose levels that are higher than normal but lower than those diagnostic for diabetes. IFG and IGT are risk factors for diabetes and cardiovascular disease. IFG is defined by a fasting plasma glucose level of 100–125 mg/dl (6.1–6.9 mmol/l); IGT is defined by a plasma glucose level 2 h after a 75-g OGTT of 140–199 mg/dl (7.8–11.0 mmol/l).

■ Gestational diabetes is defined as glucose intolerance with onset of first recognition during pregnancy. Screening for gestational diabetes is recommended for most women between the 24th and 28th week of pregnancy. Women who have a plasma glucose level of ≥140 mg/dl (≥7.8 mmol/l) 1 h after a 50-g oral glucose load should have a definitive 3-h 100-g OGTT. Some centers use ≥130 mg/dl (≥7.2 mmol/l) as the screening cut point.

Diagnosis and Classification

Diabetes represents a group of disorders associated with abnormalities in the metabolism of carbohydrate, protein, and fat and characterized by distinct eye, kidney, and nerve complications and an increased risk of cardiovascular disease. Although diabetes affects the metabolism of all body fuels, its diagnosis depends on identification of specific plasma glucose abnormalities.

A number of approaches have been used to define diabetes. Some have been based on statistical approaches to defining abnormal or high glucose levels and others on the risk of complications. In populations with a low prevalence of diabetes, glucose levels have a normal or "bell-shaped" distribution, and diabetes may be defined as glucose levels greater than the mean glucose level plus 2 standard deviations (Fig. 1.1*A*). In the 1950s, Fajans and Conn studied large groups of healthy, lean individuals without family histories of diabetes, administered oral glucose loads, and measured glucose levels at time intervals after the glucose loads. They observed normal distributions of glucose levels 60, 90, and 120 minutes after the glucose load and defined abnormal glucose tolerance based on this simple statistical approach. In populations with a high prevalence of diabetes, there is a bimodal distribution of glucose levels, and diabetes may be defined as glucose levels greater than the antimode (Fig. 1.1*B*). Bimodal glucose distributions were first described among Pima Indians, and in 1979, these data were used by the National Diabetes Data Group (NDDG) to establish the fasting and 2-h post–glucose load glucose criteria for diabetes.

Another approach to diagnosing diabetes looks at the association between glucose levels and complications (Fig. 1.1*C*). In 1997, the American Diabetes Association (ADA) Expert Committee used the associations between diabetic retinopathy and fasting glucose levels to modify the criteria for diabetes. A problem with this approach is that there appear to be different glycemic thresholds for different complications. In one study, the fasting plasma glucose threshold associated with retinopathy was between 108 and 130 mg/dl, consistent with the current diagnostic criterion for diabetes. More recently, however, the Diabetes Prevention Program Research Group reported that diabetic retinopathy was present in 7.6% of patients with impaired glucose tolerance (IGT), an intermediate level of glucose tolerance not meeting criteria for diabetes but too high to be considered normal (see below). Similarly, in a large middle-aged workforce, microalbuminuria was present in 16.1% of subjects with IGT and, in another study, distal symmetrical peripheral polyneuropathy was present in 10.0% of individuals with IGT. Perhaps

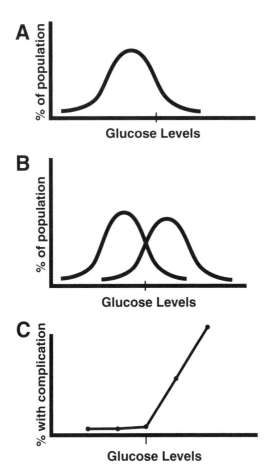

Figure 1.1 Approaches to diagnosing diabetes. *A:* Glucose level greater than the mean + 2 SDs. *B:* Glucose level more than antimode. *C:* Glucose level associated with complication.

most importantly, prospective data from nearly 30,000 patients without a history of diabetes followed for up to 11 years have demonstrated that the hazard ratio for cardiovascular mortality begins to increase with IGT.

DIAGNOSIS OF DIABETES

According to current ADA criteria, there are three ways to diagnose diabetes (Table 1.1). All require measurement of venous plasma glucose. The fasting glucose or oral glucose tolerance test (OGTT) criteria should be confirmed on a subsequent day by either of the two methods. When a subject is symptomatic and the blood glu-

Table 1.1 Criteria for the Diagnosis of Diabetes

1. Symptoms of hyperglycemia and a random plasma glucose ≥200 mg/dl (≥11.1 mmol/l). Random is defined as any time of day without regard to time since last meal. The classic symptoms of hyperglycemia include polyuria, polydipsia, and unexplained weight loss.

OR

2. Fasting plasma glucose ≥126 mg/dl (≥7.0 mmol/l). Fasting is defined as no caloric intake for at least 8 h.*

OR

3. 2-h plasma glucose ≥200 mg/dl (≥11.1 mmol/l) during an OGTT. The test should be performed as described by the WHO, using a glucose load containing the equivalent of 75 g anhydrous glucose dissolved in water.*

*In the absence of unequivocal hyperglycemia, these criteria should be confirmed by repeat testing on a different day.

cose is unequivocally elevated, the diagnosis of diabetes presents no difficulty. When a subject is without clinical symptoms or has equivocal symptoms, the diagnosis of diabetes may be more difficult. Biological and assay variation in fasting and post-load glucose measurements require confirmation by repeat testing.

Generally, the OGTT is performed only in subjects with elevated but non-diagnostic fasting glucose levels in whom there is a high index of suspicion for diabetes. Such a patient might, for example, have a fasting glucose of 115 mg/dl and evidence of cardiovascular disease or diffuse symmetric peripheral polyneuropathy. The OGTT is essentially never indicated in patients with symptoms and random glucose levels ≥200 mg/dl or patients with fasting glucose levels ≥126 mg/dl.

Although controversial, A1C is not recommended for the diagnosis of diabetes. A clear advantage of the A1C test is that the patient does not need to be fasting. Relative disadvantages include its greater cost compared with glucose and the fact that, in the past, there was a lack of standardization across laboratories and methods. However, in the U.S., A1C assays are now almost universally standardized to the Diabetes Control and Complications Trial assay. Although highly specific for the diagnosis of diabetes, A1C may be less sensitive than fasting glucose. In a study that examined the distributions of fasting glucose, 2-h glucose, and A1C in a large population and assessed the sensitivity of the antimode threshold when specificity was fixed at 99%, fasting glucose was 84% sensitive, 2-h post–glucose load glucose was 90% sensitive, and A1C was only 68% sensitive in diagnosing diabetes. Sensitivity and specificity would obviously depend on the cut points chosen. The Expert Panel on the Diagnosis and Classification of Diabetes will reconvene in 2008 to look at the issue of using A1C as a diagnostic test.

CLASSIFICATION OF DIABETES

Having established a diagnosis of diabetes, the next task is to classify the type. The purpose of classification is to differentiate and identify the various forms of the syndrome. The first generally accepted classification system was developed by the NDDG and published in 1979. The World Health Organization Study Group on Diabetes Mellitus endorsed the substantive recommendations of the NDDG in 1980 and 1985. These groups recognized two major forms of diabetes, which they termed insulin-dependent diabetes mellitus (IDDM, type I diabetes) and non-insulin-dependent diabetes mellitus (NIDDM, type II diabetes). In 1997, the ADA Expert Committee on the Diagnosis and Classification of Diabetes Mellitus recommended modifications to this classification system. The revised classification scheme was designed to reduce some of the confusion created by the previous scheme and to reflect both etiology and stage of disease. The terms "insulin-dependent diabetes mellitus" and "non-insulin-dependent diabetes mellitus" and their acronyms IDDM and NIDDM were eliminated, since they frequently resulted in classifying patients based on treatment rather than etiology. In addition, while the terms "type 1 diabetes" and "type 2 diabetes" were retained, Arabic numerals were recommended rather than Roman numerals to reduce confusion between numbers and the letter "i."

Type 1 diabetes encompasses the majority of cases that are due to pancreatic β-cell destruction and are prone to ketoacidosis. This form includes both cases ascribable to an autoimmune process and those for which an etiology is unknown. The former are defined as type 1, immune-mediated, and the latter as type 1, idiopathic. Type 2 diabetes continues to be used to describe cases in which diabetes results from insulin resistance with an insulin secretory defect. In addition, the classification system recognizes eight other specific types of diabetes (Table 1.2).

TYPE 1 DIABETES

Type 1 immune-mediated diabetes results from cell-mediated autoimmune destruction of the β-cells of the pancreatic islets. Markers of this process include islet cell autoantibodies, autoantibodies to insulin, and autoantibodies to glutamic acid decarboxylase (GAD) as well as others. One or more autoantibodies is present in up to 90% of individuals with type 1 immune-mediated diabetes at diagnosis. Patients with this form of diabetes are prone to other autoimmune disorders including Hashimoto's thyroiditis, Grave's disease, Addison's disease, pernicious anemia, and vitiligo. Type 1 immune-mediated diabetes has strong HLA associations that can be either predisposing or protective.

Immune-mediated type 1 diabetes commonly has onset in childhood and adolescence but can occur at any age. In this form of diabetes, the rate of β-cell destruction is quite variable. In general, it is more rapid in infants and children and slower in adults. This probably explains why infants and children may present with ketoacidosis as the first manifestation of disease, whereas adults may retain residual β-cell function sufficient to prevent ketoacidosis for many years. Although patients are typically not obese when they present with this type of diabetes, the presence of obesity is not incompatible with the diagnosis. In the late stages of type 1 immune-mediated diabetes, there is little or no insulin secretion, as manifested by low or undetectable levels of plasma C-peptide.

Some type 1 diabetic patients have permanent insulinopenia and are prone to ketoacidosis but have no evidence of autoimmunity. This form of diabetes, termed "idiopathic type 1 diabetes," is strongly inherited but lacks immunological evidence

Table 1.2 Etiologic Classification of Diabetes

I. Type 1 diabetes* (β-cell destruction, usually leading to absolute insulin deficiency)
   A. Immune-mediated
   B. Idiopathic
II. Type 2 diabetes* (may range from predominantly insulin resistance with relative insulin deficiency to a predominantly secretory defect with insulin resistance)
III. Other specific types
   A. Genetic defects of β-cell function
      1. Chromosome 12, HNF-1α (formerly MODY3)
      2. Chromosome 7, glucokinase (formerly MODY2)
      3. Chromosome 20, HNF-4α (formerly MODY1)
      4. Chromosome 13, insulin promoter factor-1 (IPF-1; MODY4)
      5. Chromosome 17, HNF-1β (MODY5)
      6. Chromosome 2, *NeuroD1* (MODY6)
      7. Mitochondrial DNA
      8. Others
   B. Genetic defects in insulin action
      1. Type A insulin resistance
      2. Leprechaunism
      3. Rabson-Mendenhall syndrome
      4. Lipoatrophic diabetes
      5. Others
   C. Diseases of the exocrine pancreas
      1. Pancreatitis
      2. Trauma/pancreatectomy
      3. Neoplasia
      4. Cystic fibrosis
      5. Hemochromatosis
      6. Fibrocalculous pancreatopathy
      7. Others
   D. Endocrinopathies
      1. Acromegaly
      2. Cushing's syndrome
      3. Glucagonoma
      4. Pheochromocytoma
      5. Hyperthyroidism
      6. Somatostatinoma
      7. Aldosteronoma
      8. Others
   E. Drug- or chemical-induced
      1. Vacor
      2. Pentamidine
      3. Nicotinic acid
      4. Glucocorticoids
      5. Thyroid hormone
      6. Diazoxide
      7. β-Adrenergic agonists
      8. Thiazides
      9. Dilantin
      10. α-Interferon
      11. Others
   F. Infections
      1. Congenital rubella
      2. Cytomegalovirus
      3. Others
   G. Uncommon forms of immune-mediated diabetes
      1. "Stiff-man" syndrome
      2. Anti-insulin receptor antibodies
      3. Others
   H. Other genetic syndromes sometimes associated with diabetes
      1. Down's syndrome
      2. Klinefelter's syndrome
      3. Turner's syndrome
      4. Wolfram's syndrome
      5. Friedreich's ataxia
      6. Huntington's chorea
      7. Lawrence Moon Beidel syndrome
      8. Myotonic dystrophy
      9. Porphyria
      10. Prader-Willi syndrome
      11. Others
IV. GDM

*Patients with any form of diabetes may require insulin treatment at some stage of their disease. Such use of insulin does not, of itself, classify the patient.

for β-cell autoimmunity and is not HLA associated. Individuals with this form of diabetes suffer from episodic ketoacidosis and exhibit varying degrees of insulin deficiency between episodes. Most patients with idiopathic type 1 diabetes are of African or Asian origin. An absolute requirement for insulin replacement therapy in affected patients may come and go.

TYPE 2 DIABETES

Type 2 diabetes is characterized by both impairment of insulin secretion and defects in insulin action and it is often unclear which abnormality is the primary cause of hyperglycemia. Although patients with this type of diabetes may have insulin levels that appear normal or elevated, insulin levels are always low relative to the elevated plasma glucose levels. Thus, insulin secretion is defective in these patients and insufficient to compensate for the degree of insulin resistance. Although the specific etiology of type 2 diabetes is unknown, autoimmune destruction of β-cells does not occur. Although type 2 diabetes is associated with a strong genetic predisposition, the genetics of this form of diabetes are complex and not clearly defined.

The risk of type 2 diabetes increases with age, obesity, and physical inactivity. Although type 1 diabetes remains the most common type of diabetes in children and adolescents, type 2 diabetes now accounts for one-quarter to one-third of diabetes in ages 10–19 years, particularly in racial and ethnic minority populations. Patients with type 2 diabetes who are not obese by traditional weight criteria may have an increased percentage of body fat distributed predominantly in the abdominal region. Type 2 diabetes occurs more frequently in women with prior gestational diabetes and in individuals with hypertension and dyslipidemia. Its frequency varies in different racial and ethnic groups. The traditional thinking is that ketoacidosis seldom occurs spontaneously in type 2 diabetes but may arise in association with the stress of another illness. However, there are increasing reports of patients who present with ketoacidosis but subsequently have a clear phenotype of type 2 diabetes, including long-term insulin independence.

OTHER SPECIFIC TYPES OF DIABETES

In the current classification scheme, the class of other specific types of diabetes includes eight categories: those associated with genetic defects of β-cell function, genetic defects in insulin action, diseases of the exocrine pancreas, endocrinopathies, drug- or chemical-induced diabetes, infections, uncommon forms of immune-mediated diabetes, and other genetic syndromes sometimes associated with diabetes. These categories include the fewest patients and may represent <3% of all people with diabetes. Nevertheless, correct identification of these patients is important because their treatment and prognosis may differ. Recognition of patients with other specific types of diabetes requires clinical alertness to identify the history or physical features that lead to the correct diagnosis.

STAGE OF DISEASE

In addition to reflecting etiology, the ADA classification system reflects stage of disease (Fig. 1.2). Regardless of the type of diabetes and underlying patho-

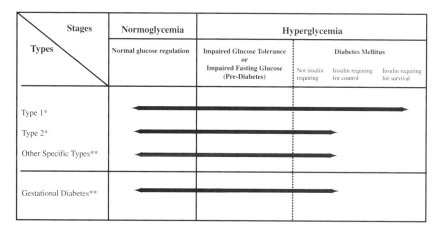

Types \ Stages	Normoglycemia	Hyperglycemia			
	Normal glucose regulation	Impaired Glucose Tolerance or Impaired Fasting Glucose (Pre-Diabetes)	Diabetes Mellitus		
			Not insulin requiring	Insulin requiring for control	Insulin requiring for survival
Type 1*					
Type 2*					
Other Specific Types**					
Gestational Diabetes**					

Figure 1.2 Disorders of glycemia: etiologic types and stages. *Even after presenting in ketoacidosis, these patients can briefly return to normoglycemia without requiring continuous therapy (i.e., "honeymoon" remission). **In rare instances, patients in these categories (e.g., Vacor toxicity, type 1 diabetes presenting in pregnancy) may require insulin for survival.

physiological mechanism, the degree of hyperglycemia (if any) may change over time. A disease process may be present but may not have progressed far enough to cause any hyperglycemia. The same disease process can cause hyperglycemia that is not sufficient to fulfill the criteria for the diagnosis of diabetes. Other individuals with type 1 immune-mediated diabetes but with residual β-cell function may not require exogenous insulin for adequate glycemic control. The severity of the metabolic abnormality can progress, regress, or stay the same. Thus, the degree of hyperglycemia reflects the severity of the underlying disease process more than the nature of the process itself. Thus, classification of type of diabetes can be made independent of stage.

SCREENING FOR DIABETES

Approximately one-third of Americans with diabetes remain undiagnosed. Screening for diabetes has been recommended to identify individuals with previously undiagnosed diabetes so that they may receive appropriate medical care. Support for diabetes screening is not based on randomized controlled clinical trials but on observational studies that have found that people diagnosed with diabetes as a result of screening have lower A1C levels and better outcomes than those presenting spontaneously with diabetes. The ADA recommends that at-risk individuals be screened periodically for diabetes as a part of their routine medical care (opportunistic screening). Few, if any, organizations recommend population screening.

Although much attention has focused on the need to increase screening rates, most patients within primary care already have periodic assessments of glycemia. In one study of a large managed care organization, 69% of nondiabetic members ≥45 years of age had received at least one test of glycemia in the previous 3 years. The frequency of testing increased with age, non-white race, overweight or obesity, hypertension, dyslipidemia, family history of diabetes, and previous diagnosis of abnormal glucose tolerance. Random glucose was the most common screening method (95%). Only a minority of patients were screened with fasting glucose or OGTT.

Unfortunately, because the random glucose level diagnostic of diabetes (in association with symptoms) is ≥200 mg/dl, many patients without symptoms but with elevated but non-diagnostic random glucose levels do not undergo further diagnostic testing. Studies examining random glucose as a screening test for diabetes have demonstrated that a random glucose ≥130 mg/dl provides optimal sensitivity and specificity as a screening test for diabetes. All random glucose levels ≥130 mg/dl must be followed up with a definitive diagnostic test as outlined above. Simulation models have suggested that use of a random glucose test every 3 years with a cut point for an abnormal test of 130 mg/dl provides a good yield and minimizes the number of false-positive screening tests requiring follow-up.

There has also been interest in developing multivariate models to screen for diabetes. These have included equations to predict future risk of diabetes and equations to predict prevalent undiagnosed diabetes. Investigators have used Egyptian populations, Dutch populations, English, Danish, and Indian populations to develop these screening models. In general, equations that do not include glucose measures have not performed as well as those that have in predicting prevalent undiagnosed diabetes.

IGT AND IMPAIRED FASTING GLUCOSE

Individuals with IGT or impaired fasting glucose (IFG) have glucose levels higher than normal but lower than those diagnostic of diabetes. IGT is diagnosed by the 2-h 75-g OGTT, where fasting glucose is <126 mg/dl and 2-h glucose is between 140 and 199 mg/dl. IGT is a risk factor for diabetes and cardiovascular disease. In general, the incidence of type 2 diabetes in individuals with IGT is 5% per year with a range from 4 to 9% per year. Risk factors for progression include higher 2-h post–glucose load glucose levels and Hispanic and Native American ethnicity. Individuals with IGT have a risk of cardiovascular disease and cardiovascular mortality approximately twofold higher than individuals with normal glucose tolerance and similar to individuals with type 2 diabetes.

The ADA's decision to focus on the fasting glucose as the primary diagnostic test for diabetes made it less likely that patients would be diagnosed with IGT. In an effort to rectify this problem, the ADA created a new classification of glucose intolerance termed "impaired fasting glucose." In 1997, IFG was defined as a fasting glucose of 110–125 mg/dl. Subsequent studies demonstrated that people with IFG had an increased risk for progression to type 2 diabetes and an increased risk of cardiovascular disease. The World Health Organization (WHO) subsequently endorsed this classification of IFG in 1999. In 2003, the ADA recognized that fewer individuals were diagnosed with IFG than IGT and therefore lowered the diagnostic criterion for IFG to 100–125 mg/dl. Although this change increased the numbers of people diagnosed with IFG, subjects diagnosed with IFG with fasting glucose levels between 100 and 110 mg/dl are different from subjects with IGT and, in general, are at lower risk for both diabetes and cardiovascular disease. The WHO has declined to endorse this modification and continues to diagnose IFG on the basis of a fasting glucose between 110 and 125 mg/dl.

GESTATIONAL DIABETES

Gestational diabetes mellitus (GDM) is defined as glucose intolerance with onset or first recognition during pregnancy. GDM affects ~4% of pregnancies, or about 200,000 American women each year. Diagnostic criteria for GDM were initially developed to predict future maternal risk of type 2 diabetes. Approximately 5–10% of women with GDM are diagnosed with type 2 diabetes in the postpartum period, and up to 50% develop type 2 diabetes within 10 years. Treatment is now largely focused on glycemic control to prevent fetal macrosomia. Both the size of the baby and need for a first cesarean delivery are related to the degree of maternal hyperglycemia, and treatment reduces the risk of these adverse outcomes.

Screening for GDM is recommended for most pregnant women (Table 1.3). Assessment of risk for GDM should be performed at the first prenatal visit, and women at very high risk should be screened immediately using a random, fasting, or post–glucose load glucose level. Most women not found to have GDM should undergo further screening at 24–28 weeks of gestation. In lower-risk women, the glucose level is measured 1 h after a 50-g oral glucose load without regard to the time of day or time of last food. A value ≥130 mg/dl has 90% sensitivity for detecting GDM and a value ≥140 mg/dl has an 80% sensitivity for detecting GDM by the "gold standard" 3-h 100-g OGTT. In higher-risk women, including those with previous histories of GDM, the diagnostic 3-h 100-g OGTT should be performed without first performing the 50-g screening test.

Because women with histories of GDM are at increased risk for postpartum diabetes, they should be retested after delivery. The Fifth International Workshop–Conference on Gestational Diabetes recommended measuring fasting or random glucose levels before discharge from the hospital and performing a 2-h 75-g OGTT at 6–12 weeks after delivery. A repeat OGTT is recommended at 1 year and, at a minimum, every 3 years thereafter.

RISK FACTOR CLUSTERING

Hyperglycemia and type 2 diabetes cluster with a number of other cardiovascular risk factors. Syndrome X, originally described by Reaven, included insulin resistance, hyperinsulinemia, glucose intolerance, increased triglycerides, decreased HDL cholesterol, and hypertension. More recent descriptions of the cluster also include increased body weight (especially central adiposity), inflammation, microalbuminuria, hyperuricemia, and abnormalities of coagulation and fibrinolysis. In most instances, excess nutrition and associated insulin resistance likely underlies many of these metabolic abnormalities, although some individuals with these risk factors do not manifest insulin resistance.

Table 1.3 Screening for and Diagnosis of GDM

Carry out GDM risk assessment at the first prenatal visit.
Women at very high risk for GDM should be screened for diabetes as soon as possible after the confirmation of pregnancy. Criteria for very high risk are:

- Severe obesity
- Prior history of GDM or delivery of large-for-gestational-age infant
- Presence of glycosuria
- Diagnosis of polycystic ovarian syndrome
- Strong family history of type 2 diabetes

Screening/diagnosis at this stage of pregnancy should use standard diagnostic testing. All women of higher than low risk of GDM, including those above not found to have diabetes early in pregnancy, should undergo GDM testing at 24–28 weeks of gestation. Low risk status, which does not require GDM screening, is defined as women with *all* of the following characteristics:

- Age <25 years
- Weight normal before pregnancy
- Member of an ethnic group with a low prevalence of diabetes
- No known diabetes in first-degree relatives
- No history of abnormal glucose tolerance
- No history of poor obstetrical outcome

Two approaches may be followed for GDM screening at 24–28 weeks:

1. Two-step approach:
   a. Perform initial screening by measuring plasma or serum glucose 1 h after a 50-g oral glucose load. A glucose threshold after a 50-g load of ≥140 mg/dl identifies ~80% of women with GDM, whereas the sensitivity is further increased to ~90% by a threshold of ≥130 mg/dl.
   b. Perform a diagnostic 100-g OGTT on a separate day in women who exceed the chosen threshold on 50-g screening.
2. One-step approach (may be preferred in clinics with high prevalence of GDM): Perform a diagnostic 100-g OGTT in all women to be tested at 24–28 weeks.

The 100-g OGTT should be performed in the morning after an overnight fast of at least 8 h. A diagnosis of GDM requires at least two of the following plasma glucose values:

Fasting: ≥95 mg/dl (≥5.3 mmol/l)
1 h: ≥180 mg/dl (≥10.0 mmol/l)
2 h: ≥155 mg/dl (≥8.6 mmol/l)
3 h: ≥140 mg/dl (≥7.8 mmol/l)

The cluster of phenotypic abnormalities came to be termed the metabolic syndrome, and clearly individuals with the metabolic syndrome are at risk for type 2 diabetes and cardiovascular disease. There is no uniform definition of the metabolic syndrome, but there are similarities between the criteria proposed by the U.S. Expert Panel on Detection, Evaluation, and Treatment of High Blood Cholesterol in Adults (Adult Treatment Panel III [ATP III]) and the WHO, with both including the presence of at least three of five abnormalities encompassing adiposity, dyslipidemia, hypertension, and hyperglycemia. Data from the Third National Health and Nutrition Examination Survey (NHANES III), which used the ATP III criteria, found that the prevalence of the metabolic syndrome in the U.S. was ~20–25%. The prevalence of the metabolic syndrome increases with age and is highest in Latino populations, affecting up to 50% of adults 40–74 years of age.

Recent concerns surrounding the term metabolic syndrome as a distinct clinical entity have not disputed the clustering of cardiovascular risk factors including central obesity, dyslipidemia, and hypertension, nor the association of the metabolic syndrome with the risk of diabetes and cardiovascular disease. Instead, the controversy has focused on the etiology of the syndrome, its somewhat arbitrary definition, and how clinical decision-making would be modified based on a diagnosis of metabolic syndrome compared with appropriate treatment of each risk factor. The risks of diabetes and cardiovascular disease imparted by the metabolic syndrome seem to be explained by the risks of the individual components.

EVALUATION AND CLASSIFICATION OF PATIENTS BEFORE TREATMENT

Before therapy is initiated to treat diabetes, the patient should have a complete medical evaluation. The complete medical evaluation helps the physician classify the patient, detect the presence of complications frequently associated with diabetes (see Chapter 5), ascertain the presence of comorbid diseases, and provide the basis for formulating a management plan. Table 1.4 provides an outline for the initial medical evaluation.

Usually, a reasonably good initial classification of the patient can be made on the basis of a complete personal and family history and the diagnostic test results. Patients should not be classified on the basis of age alone or on whether they are taking insulin. If the diagnosis of diabetes had been made previously, an initial evaluation should also review the previous treatment and the past and present degrees of glycemic control. Laboratory tests appropriate to the evaluation of each patient's general medical condition should be performed.

A major problem in classification is that it is sometimes difficult to assign the patient to a particular type of diabetes (i.e., type 1 or type 2). For example, the normal-weight patient with type 2 diabetes who has been taking insulin may appear to have type 1 diabetes. Some patients with type 2 diabetes require insulin for glycemic control but do not depend on insulin to prevent ketoacidosis or to sustain life. Another example is the newly diagnosed child or adolescent who is a member of a family with an autosomal-dominant form of diabetes such as maturity-onset diabetes of the young (MODY). The family history will provide the clue to the correct diagnosis. Such a patient should not be classified as having type 1 diabetes on the basis of age alone. Other patients, particularly adults, have type 1 immune-mediated diabetes but are at a stage in which they still have β-cell function and clinically appear similar to individuals with type 2 diabetes. Finally, the emerging recognition of ketosis-prone type 2 diabetes, especially in young adult African-American or Latino patients, can make classification initially confusing. It usually is not necessary for clinicians to determine the presence of islet cell or other antibodies or the degree of insulin secretion, but in ketosis-prone diabetes, these measurements may be helpful.

Table 1.4 Initial Medical Evaluation for the Patient with Diabetes

Medical History

- Age and characteristics of onset of diabetes (e.g., diabetic ketoacidosis, asymptomatic laboratory finding)
- Family history of diabetes
- Eating patterns, nutritional status, and weight history; growth and development in children and adolescents
- Diabetes education history
- Review of previous treatment regimens and response to therapy (A1C records)
- Current treatment of diabetes, including medications, meal plan, physical activity patterns, and results of glucose monitoring and patient's use of data
- Diabetic ketoacidosis frequency, severity, and cause
  - Hypoglycemia awareness
  - Any severe hypoglycemia: frequency and cause
- History of diabetes-related complications
  - Microvascular: retinopathy, nephropathy, neuropathy (sensory, including history of foot lesions; autonomic, including sexual dysfunction and gastroparesis)
  - Macrovascular: coronary heart disease, cerebrovascular disease, peripheral arterial disease
  - Other: psychosocial problems, dental disease
- Other endocrine disorders

Physical Examination

- Height, weight, BMI
- Blood pressure determination, including orthostatic measurements when indicated
- Fundoscopic examination*
- Thyroid palpation

- Skin examination (for acanthosis nigricans and insulin injection sites)
- Complete foot examination
  - Inspection
  - Palpation of dorsalis pedis and posterior tibial pulses
  - Presence/absence of patellar and Achilles reflexes
  - Determination of proprioception, vibration, and monofilament sensation

Laboratory Evaluation

- A1C, if results are not available within the past 2–3 months

If not performed/available within past year

- Fasting lipid profile, including total, LDL, and HDL cholesterol and triglycerides
- Liver function tests
- Tests for urine albumin excretion with spot urine albumin-to-creatinine ratio
- Serum creatinine and calculated glomerular filtration rate
- Thyroid-stimulating hormone in all type 1 diabetic subjects, dyslipidemic patients, or women over age 50

Referrals

- Annual dilated eye exam
- Family planning for women of reproductive age
- Registered dietitian for medical nutrition therapy
- Diabetes self-management education
- Dental examination
- Mental health professional, if needed

*See appropriate referrals for these categories.

BIBLIOGRAPHY

American Diabetes Association: Diagnosis and classification of diabetes mellitus. *Diabetes Care* 31:S55–S60, 2008

Baan CA, Ruige JB, Stolk RP, Witteman JCM, Dekker JM, Heine RJ, Feskens EJM: Performance of a predictive model to identify undiagnosed diabetes in a health care setting. *Diabetes Care* 22:213–219, 1999

Balasubramanyam A, Garza G, Rodriguez L, Hampe CS, Gaur L, Lernmark A, Maldonado MR: Accuracy and predictive value of classification schemes for ketosis-prone diabetes. *Diabetes Care* 29:2575–2579, 2006

Ealovega MW, Tabaei BP, Brandle M, Burke R, Herman WH: Opportunistic screening for diabetes in routine clinical practice. *Diabetes Care* 27:9–12, 2004

Engelgau MM, Venkat Narayan KM, Herman WH: Screening for type 2 diabetes. *Diabetes Care* 23:1563–1580, 2000

Expert Committee on the Diagnosis and Classification of Diabetes Mellitus: Report of the Expert Committee on the Diagnosis and Classification of Diabetes Mellitus. *Diabetes Care* 20:1183–1197, 1997

Ford ES, Giles WH: A comparison of the prevalence of the metabolic syndrome using two proposed definitions. *Diabetes Care* 26:575–581, 2003

Glumer C, Carstensen B, Sandbaek A, Lauritzen T, Jorgensen T, Borch-Johnsen K: A Danish diabetes risk score for targeted screening: The Inter99 Study. *Diabetes Care* 27:727–733, 2004

Griffin SJ, Little PS, Hales CN, Kinmonth AL, Wareham NJ: Diabetes risk score: towards earlier detection of type 2 diabetes in general practice. *Diabetes Metab Res Rev* 16:164–171, 2000

Herman WH: Diabetes epidemiology: guiding clinical and public health practice. *Diabetes Care* 30:1912–1919, 2007

Johnson SL, Tabaei BP, Herman WH: The efficacy and cost of alternative strategies for systematic screening for type 2 diabetes in the US population 45–74 years of age. *Diabetes Care* 28:307–311, 2005

Kahn R, Buse J, Ferrannini E, Stern M, American Diabetes Association, European Association for the Study of Diabetes: The metabolic syndrome: time for a critical appraisal: joint statement from the American Diabetes Association and the European Association for the Study of Diabetes. *Diabetes Care* 28:2289–2304, 2005

National Diabetes Data Group: Classification and diagnosis of diabetes mellitus and other categories of glucose intolerance. *Diabetes* 28:1039–1057, 1979

Ramachandran A, Snehalatha C, Vijay V, Wareham NJ, Colaguiri S: Derivation and validation of diabetes risk score for urban Asian Indians. *Diabetes Res Clin Pract* 70:63–70, 2005

SEARCH for Diabetes in Youth Study Group: Incidence of diabetes in youth in the United States. *JAMA* 297:2716–2724, 2007

Tabaei BP, Herman WH: A multivariate logistic regression equation to screen for diabetes: development and validation. *Diabetes Care* 25:1999–2003, 2002

World Health Organization: *WHO Expert Committee on Diabetes Mellitus: Second Report.* Geneva, World Health Org., 1980 (Tech. Rep. Ser., no. 646)

World Health Organization: *Diabetes Mellitus: Report of a WHO Study Group.* Geneva, World Health Org., 1985 (Tech. Rep. Ser., no. 727)

Pathogenesis

Highlights
Pathogenesis

■ Most type 2 diabetes develops in obese individuals who have a genetic predisposition to β-cell failure.

■ A monogenetic cause of diabetes has been identified in only a small fraction of individuals with type 2 diabetes. A number of genes that contribute to the risk have been identified. Likely, the genetic risk is produced by the interaction of multiple genes, each of which confers an incremental risk for the development of the disease.

■ Defects in insulin action and insulin secretion are seen in most individuals with type 2 diabetes.

■ Skeletal muscle, liver, and adipose tissue are the primary sites of insulin resistance.

■ β-Cell dysfunction, leading to a relative decrease in insulin levels, is a progressive process and likely results from intrinsic secretion failure and decreases in β-cell mass.

■ Abnormalities in the uptake and metabolism of fatty acid in peripheral tissues and in the β-cells may be a primary event in the development of insulin resistance and β-cell failure.

■ Inflammatory responses of tissue to excess nutrients may contribute to the insulin resistance found in type 2 diabetes.

Pathogenesis

Type 2 diabetes is a chronic disorder characterized by diminished liver, muscle, and adipose tissue sensitivity to insulin, termed "insulin resistance," and a superimposed impairment of β-cell secretory function. Although abnormal carbohydrate metabolism is the defining disorder, changes in fat and protein metabolism clearly occur and contribute to the complications arising from this progressive metabolic disease. Type 2 diabetes is the most common form of diabetes, accounting for >90% of cases. In most cases, the development of type 2 diabetes is due to environmental influences on a susceptible genetic background. Worldwide, the incidence of diabetes is rising rapidly because of modernization and the resultant access to greater quantities of foodstuffs and modern conveniences that lead to increased caloric consumption and decreased energy expenditure.

GENETIC AND ENVIRONMENTAL FACTORS

Multiple lines of evidence show that type 2 diabetes is a genetic disease. The incidence of type 2 diabetes is especially high among certain ethnic populations such as Hispanics/Latinos, Aboriginal peoples in the Americas and Australia, Pacific and Indian Ocean island populations, and the peoples of the Indian subcontinent. A family history of type 2 diabetes is another important risk factor for the development of diabetes. Specific genetic aberrations are present in only small subpopulations with type 2 diabetes, such as those seen in maturity-onset diabetes of the young (MODY).

Additional candidate gene studies have identified the E23K variant in the potassium inwardly rectifying channel, subfamily J, member 11 (KCNJ11); the P12A variant in the peroxisome proliferator–activated receptor-γ (*PPARG*) gene; common variation in the transcription factor 2, hepatic (TCF2); and the Wolfram syndrome 1 (WFS1). Recent genome-wide scans have identified variations in several additional genes that show a statistically significant association with risk for type 2 diabetes. These include CDKAL1 (CDK5 regulatory subunit–associated protein 1–like 1), CDKN2 (cyclin-dependent kinase inhibitor 2A), FTO (fat mass and obesity–associated), HHEX (hematopoietically expressed homeobox), IDE (insulin-degrading enzyme), and IGF2BP2 (insulin-like growth factor 2 mRNA-binding protein 2). It is likely that variation in the structure or expression of other genes will be identified that modulate the risk for type 2 diabetes.

For most individuals, the genetic risk is likely due to interactions between several genes, each of which can protect or sensitize an individual to the consequence of increased food intake and decreased physical activity. The way in which these genetic variations interact to predispose an individual to diabetes has not been determined. With the identification of rare forms of type 2 diabetes and genes that confer risk, several companies are offering tests may predict increased genetic susceptibility to type 2 diabetes. However, with the exception of the rare monogenic forms of diabetes, the clinical utility of these tests is not apparent.

The genes that predispose an individual to diabetes have likely been selected through evolution. Until recently, humans lived in a relatively nutrient-poor environment. Possessing genes that allow for the efficient accumulation and storage of nutrients would be a distinct advantage during times of chronic or intermittent food shortage. However, these so-called "thrifty genes" are maladaptive in today's consistently food-rich environment.

At present, there is no clear indication that ingestion of a certain type of nutrient, whether carbohydrate, fat, or protein, independent of total caloric intake, is more harmful with respect to the development of diabetes. The combination of a sedentary lifestyle with an increased caloric intake leading to weight gain and the development of obesity is the primary factor in the development of insulin resistance and ultimately type 2 diabetes.

INSULIN RESISTANCE

Insulin resistance is defined as a decrease in the activity of endogenous or exogenously administered insulin to alter metabolism in target tissues. Insulin resistance is a consistent finding in patients with type 2 diabetes, and resistance is present years before the onset of diabetes and predicts the onset of diabetes. Most individuals are able to maintain normal glucose levels by increasing β-cell insulin production to compensate for the decrease in insulin action. However, in susceptible individuals, increasing insulin resistance or a failure of β-cells to maintain high levels of insulin secretion leads to progressive glucose intolerance and subsequent diabetes. It is likely that genetic factors play a role both in the propensity to develop insulin resistance and in the risk for β-cell failure in response to insulin resistance.

SITES OF INSULIN RESISTANCE

Insulin resistance exists in both hepatic and peripheral tissues. Skeletal muscle is the primary site of glucose uptake after a meal and is the primary site of insulin resistance. Decreases in skeletal muscle glucose uptake and nonoxidative disposal (predominantly glycogen synthesis) are the main findings in diabetes. The decrease in insulin-mediated muscle glucose disposal contributes to the excessive rise in plasma glucose concentration after a mixed meal in patients with type 2 diabetes. Adipose tissue also shows resistance to insulin-stimulated glucose uptake as well as resistance to inhibition of lipolysis.

In the liver, insulin resistance leads to a failure to suppress hepatic glucose production, even in the face of fasting hyperinsulinemia. Basal rates of hepatic glucose production are increased when the fasting plasma glucose exceeds 110 mg/dl (6.1 mmol/l). Increases in hepatic glucose production directly correlate with the level of fasting plasma glucose. Patients with type 2 diabetes do not demonstrate normal suppression of hepatic glucose output when insulin is infused intravenously at a low concentration. At high infusion concentrations of insulin, hepatic glucose output can be suppressed, indicating partial ability to overcome the insulin resistance.

MECHANISMS OF INSULIN RESISTANCE

The action of insulin on its target tissues is influenced by sex, age, ethnicity, physical activity, medications, and, most importantly, weight. Insulin resistance is known to be present to some degree in most obese individuals and is found in most individuals with type 2 diabetes. It is important to realize that not all obese individuals develop insulin resistance for reasons that remain unclear. However, in general, the degree of obesity, as manifested by BMI, correlates well with the degree of insulin resistance and with the risk for type 2 diabetes. The relationship between BMI and diabetes risk is different among ethnic populations. For example, the risk for diabetes occurs at a lower BMI in Asian individuals than in most other ethnic groups.

The development of obesity commonly results in an accumulation of intra-abdominal fat, which may be a stronger predictor of type 2 diabetes than overall BMI. Intra-abdominal fat is metabolically distinct from subcutaneous fat. It is more lipolytically active and less sensitive to the antilipolytic effects of insulin. This results in increases in the flux of free fatty acids (FFAs) from the fat to the liver and to the periphery. Despite increased flux, serum FFAs may not be markedly elevated because of efficient extraction by the liver and skeletal muscle. Excess delivery of FFAs stimulates liver glucose production, decreases skeletal muscle insulin sensitivity, and results in blunted insulin release as well as affected vascular reactivity and coagulation parameters. Inflammatory response is a consistent finding in muscle and other tissues exposed to increases in nutrient fluxes. The inflammatory response may both initiate the insulin resistance in a tissue and result in elaboration of additional inflammatory molecules, resulting in greater resistance.

The cellular processes that are affected in the muscle, liver, and β-cells leading to insulin resistance are becoming clarified, but the exact mechanisms remain to be determined. In muscle, a small reduction in insulin binding to its cell surface receptor is observed in type 2 diabetes and is caused by downregulation of the receptor in response to hyperinsulinemia. Although abnormal insulin binding associated with rare mutations in the insulin gene and the insulin receptor result in significant insulin resistance, it is not thought that the abnormalities associated with type 2 diabetes are of sufficient magnitude to result in the degree of insulin resistance commonly seen.

Post-receptor abnormalities are primarily responsible for insulin resistance in the skeletal muscle and liver in patients with type 2 diabetes. After binding insulin, the insulin receptor initiates a complex cascade of protein phosphorylations and dephosphorylations and other processes that result in various cellular events. Increases, decreases, and aberrant phosphorylation of specific proteins, including the insulin receptor, result in impaired propagation of signals. This decreases the translocation of the glucose transporter proteins from the cytoplasm to the cell membrane, resulting in decreased glucose transport and activation of glycogen synthesis and impaired mitochondrial oxidation of substrates.

In the liver, elevated FFAs may antagonize the effects of insulin to suppress endogenous glucose production. There is a direct relationship between the fasting blood glucose and the resistance of the liver to insulin. Peripheral insulin resistance may also play a role in the increased glucose production by the liver. The inability of insulin to suppress the mobilization of gluconeogenic precursors from peripheral tissue results in their increased delivery to the liver and stimulation of gluconeogenesis.

In both muscle and liver, the accumulation of intracellular stores of triglyceride strongly correlates with the degree of insulin resistance. This accumulation is likely a marker of an inequality of fatty acid delivery (or synthesis in the liver) and the ability of these tissues to oxidize the fats. This leads to the buildup of long-chain acyl-CoA molecules, which can act as signaling molecules. The accumulation of the acyl-CoA molecules is exacerbated by glucose and its metabolites, which can lead to decreases in fatty acid import into the mitochondria and decreasing oxidation. Recent studies in animals and in humans have provided evidence for both intrinsic (inherited) defects in mitochondrial metabolism and acquired mitochondrial changes that result in decreases in oxidation of fatty acids.

A prevailing theory for the enhanced delivery of fatty acids to peripheral tissue in insulin-resistant individuals and those with type 2 diabetes is the "overflow" hypothesis. The limited ability an individual has to expand his or her adipose mass results in the excess fatty acids "overflowing" into other tissues, disrupting their normal metabolism. An extreme example of this phenomenon is seen in individuals with lipodystrophy, who have a partial or complete absence of adipose tissue. These individuals develop extreme insulin resistance, elevated serum triglyceride and FFA levels, and accumulation of "ectopic" triglyceride stores in muscle and liver associated with steatosis, inflammation, and cirrhosis. The same clinical features are found in most individuals with type 2 diabetes, suggesting a similar pathophysiological mechanism resulting in insulin resistance.

THE FAT CELL AS AN ENDOCRINE ORGAN

Adipose tissue produces numerous proteins that act as local paracrine factors and also circulate to modulate both feeding behavior and insulin action. The most well described of these is leptin, which modulates feeding behavior through interaction with specific receptors in the brain. Besides suppressing food intake, leptin plays a role in modulating glucose and lipid metabolism in the periphery and also regulates energy expenditure. These effects are primarily through the autonomic nervous system, although some actions may be direct. In addition to leptin, the fat cell expresses adiponectin, resistin, tumor necrosis factor (TNF)-α, interleukin (IL)-6, and a variety of other proteins that alter the sensitivity of tissues to insulin and may play a role in the pathogenesis of type 2 diabetes.

Adipose tissue function can be modulated by a variety of factors, including FFAs and hormones. In addition, a number of studies have suggested that elaboration of inflammatory mediators may result in infiltration of adipose tissue with macrophages, which may exacerbate adipocyte dysfunction.

DEFECTS IN INSULIN SECRETION

Insulin sensitivity is an important factor in determining the magnitude of the insulin response to β-cell stimulation by glucose, its primary secretagogue. When β-cell function is assessed, obese people who are insulin resistant manifest greater responses than lean people. However, the pattern of insulin release is abnormal. The first phase of insulin release is blunted or absent, whereas the second phase is enhanced and prolonged, resulting in overall hyperinsulinemia. The ability of the β-cell to secrete insulin in an oscillatory manner is disrupted and the ability of the islet to secrete insulin after experimental rises in blood glucose concentrations is blunted. A defect in the normal ratio of proinsulin to insulin is observed, with decreased processing of insulin leading to relative increases in proinsulin.

At diagnosis of type 2 diabetes, ~50% of β-cell function has already been lost. With time, further deterioration occurs regardless of dietary, metformin, or sulfonylurea therapy. However, it appears that some stabilization of β-cell function can result from increasing insulin sensitivity by diet, exercise, or treatment with insulin-sensitizing drugs such as the thiazolidinediones. As a result, diabetes appears to be a progressive disorder in which secondary failure of therapeutic interventions is predictable and additional drug therapies are usually required.

In islets, FFAs are important for normal secretion of insulin, whereas excess delivery of FFAs results in a reduction in glucose-stimulated insulin release. The accumulation of long-chain acyl-CoA molecules, leading to disrupted intracellular signaling, oxidative stress, the generation of ceramides, and the accumulation of amyloid protein, have all been proposed to contribute to β-cell dysfunction.

Autopsy examinations have demonstrated the association of obesity with an increase in β-cell number, whereas individuals with established type 2 diabetes have about a 50% decrease in β-cell number, and it has been suggested that the decrease in β-cell number is the primary factor in reduction in insulin secretion. Interestingly, decreases are seen in both thin and obese individuals with type 2 diabetes. Although a longitudinal study of β-cell mass is not possible, it may be that individuals who developed diabetes have an intrinsically reduced β-cell mass that predisposed them to the disease.

FACTORS MODULATING INSULIN SECRETION

Incretin hormones (glucagon-like peptide [GLP]-1, glucose-dependent insulinotropic peptide [GIP]-1, and GIP-2) are released from small intestine endocrine cells after a meal. The proteins act directly on the β-cells to increase their sensitivity to glucose but do not stimulate insulin secretion by themselves. The "incretin" effect of these hormones likely explains the significantly larger secretion of insulin from the β-cell after oral glucose as opposed to that seen after intravenous glucose administration. Some studies suggest that a defect exists in the release and/or response of these hormones in insulin resistance and type 2 diabetes. Pharmacologic doses of the native GLP-1 peptide or biologically active analogs, such as extendin 4, can result in a significant potentiation in insulin release in both normal individuals and individuals with type 2 diabetes. This property has been exploited by recently approved incretin mimetic medications, such as exenatide and inhibitors of GLP-1 degrading dipeptidyl peptidase-4 (DPP-4). In contrast, treatment with pharmacologic doses of GIP increases insulin secretion only in individuals without diabetes.

Insulin secretion is also influenced by other gut hormones, including cholecystokinin (CCK), secretin, vasoactive intestinal polypeptide (VIP), and gastrin. What roles these hormones play in blunted insulin secretion in type 2 diabetes remains to be determined, but their effects are believed to be minor.

PHYSIOLOGICAL CONSEQUENCES OF DEFECTIVE INSULIN SECRETION

Regardless of the mechanism, the impairment in insulin secretion in type 2 diabetes after meal ingestion has physiological consequences. When the early phase of insulin secretion is reduced, portal vein insulin concentration remains low after food ingestion and hepatic glucose production is not suppressed. This effect may be exacerbated by a relative increase in glucagon secretion from islets. Continued output of glucose by the liver plus the glucose entering the circulation from the intestinal tract lead to hyperglycemia. In addition, because of the reduced insulin secretion, glucose uptake by muscle is reduced, accentuating the hyperglycemia. Early in the progression to diabetes, the reduced first-phase insulin secretion is followed by late enhanced insulin secretion. Eventually, the plasma glucose concentration returns to normal, but only at the expense of hyperglycemia and hyperinsulinemia. As the defect in β-cell insulin secretion progresses, even late insulin secretion diminishes. When this occurs, fasting hyperglycemia and overt diabetes develop.

CONCLUSION

Dual defects, insulin resistance, and a relative decrease in insulin secretion are seen in most type 2 diabetic individuals and are due to both genetic and environmental factors (Fig. 2.1). Increased insulin resistance is initially compensated for by an increase in insulin secretion, which may be due to increases in islet cell mass and increased production of insulin by individual β-cells. With a continued oversupply of nutrients relative to energy expenditure, the progressive increase in insulin resistance cannot be adequately compensated for by increased insulin secretion, resulting first in impaired glucose tolerance and then in diabetes. The cellular mechanisms resulting in muscle, liver, and adipose tissue resistance and β-cell failure may be similar, with alterations in intracellular metabolism as a result of the accumulation of excess energy manifested by increased intracellular triglyceride levels, abnormal mitochondrial function, and development of inflammation. The underlying genetic makeup of the individual dictates whether this prolonged energy imbalance results in hyperglycemia and the associated metabolic disorders associated with type 2 diabetes. Hyperglycemia and dyslipidemia themselves result in additional decreases in insulin action and insulin secretion, reinforcing the established defects in the tissues. Prevention and treatment of insulin resistance and diabetes are initially targeted to limit the positive energy balance and then to modulate the metabolic dysfunction once diabetes is established.

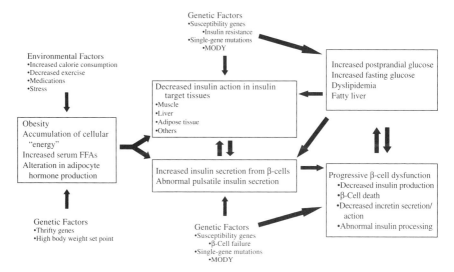

Figure 2.1 Pathogenesis of type 2 diabetes.

BIBLIOGRAPHY

Barness LA, Opitz JM, Gilbert-Barnes E: Obesity: genetic, molecular, and environmental aspects. *Am J Med Genet A* 143:3016–3034, 2007

Boden G: Pathogenesis of type 2 diabetes: insulin resistance. *Endocrinol Metab Clin North Am* 30:801–815, 2001

Boden G, Shulman G: Free fatty acids in obesity and type 2 diabetes: defining their role in the development of insulin resistance and beta-cell dysfunction. *Eur J Clin Invest* 32 (Suppl. 3):14–23, 2002

Buchanan TA: Pancreatic beta-cell loss and preservation in type 2 diabetes. *Clin Ther* 25 (Suppl. B):B32–B46, 2003

Drucker DJ, Nauck MA: The incretin system: glucagon-like peptide-1 receptor agonists and dipeptidyl peptidase-4 inhibitors in type 2 diabetes. *Lancet* 368:1696–1705, 2006

Frayling TM: Genome-wide association studies provide new insights into type 2 diabetes aetiology. *Nat Rev Genet* 8:657–662, 2007

Kahn SE: The importance of B-cell failure in the development and progression of type 2 diabetes. *J Clin Endocrinol Metab* 86:4047–4058, 2001

Petersen KF, Shulman GI: Pathogenesis of skeletal muscle insulin resistance in type 2 diabetes mellitus. *Am J Cardiol* 90:11G–18G, 2002

Pratley RE, Weyer C: The role of impaired early insulin secretion in the pathogenesis of type II diabetes mellitus. *Diabetologia* 44:929–945, 2001

Management

Assessment of Treatment Efficacy
Office methods
Self-monitoring

Highlights
Management

THERAPEUTIC OBJECTIVES AND PLAN

■ The major management goals of type 2 diabetes are to:
- Prevent microvascular and macrovascular complications
- Avoid symptoms related to adverse events of medications, hyperglycemia, and its complications

■ Specific goals of therapy are to:
- Eliminate symptoms
- Optimize glycemic parameters
- Achieve and maintain a reasonable body weight
- Achieve and maintain blood pressure control
- Achieve and maintain optimal lipoproteoprotein parameters
- Identify, prevent, and treat microvascular and macrovascular complications
- Achieve optimal overall health and well-being

■ Recommended treatment modalities include:
- Diet modification to improve glucose and lipid parameters and achieve desired body weight
- Exercise to improve glucose control and improve cardiovascular health
- Pharmacologic intervention

■ Therapy should be individualized, based on patient age, comorbidities, lifestyle, financial restrictions, self-management skills learned, and level of patient motivation.

■ Recommendations for metabolic control are found in Table 3.1.

■ Patient education that enhances self-care behaviors is essential for the successful management of type 2 diabetes.

NUTRITION

■ Medical nutrition therapy is an important element in the therapeutic plan for patients with type 2 diabetes. For some, nutrition and exercise are the only interventions needed to control the metabolic abnormalities associated with type 2 diabetes, including hyperglycemia, dyslipidemia, and hypertension.

■ When the person with diabetes is overweight, total caloric intake should be decreased to produce lasting weight loss. Caloric restriction itself is usually successful in lowering plasma glucose levels even before substantial weight loss is achieved. Approaches to weight reduction are outlined under the topic "Overweight."

■ Patients with type 2 diabetes who are of normal weight should eat sufficient calories to maintain that weight and should distribute nutrient intake throughout the day to optimize blood glucose control.

■ Recommendations for nutrient content of the diet, including fat, protein, carbohydrates, sugar and fat substitutes, and micronutrients, are presented under the topic "Protein."

■ The use of alcohol is discussed under the topic "Alcohol."

■ Successful implementation of lifestyle interventions in diabetes and pre-diabetes generally requires the guidance of health care professionals with appropriate training, usually registered dietitians with experience in behavioral modification and sensitivity to ethnic and cultural issues.

■ Successful implementation of a specific nutrition plan requires:
• Patient education and behavior modification
• Individualization of the meal plan
• Early intervention and continuous follow-up

EXERCISE

■ Unless contraindicated, appropriate physical activity is strongly recommended to maximize the effects of dietary modification.

■ The potential benefits of increased physical activity include:
• Improved insulin sensitivity and glucose tolerance
• Weight loss and maintenance of desirable body weight when combined with restricted caloric intake

• Improved cardiovascular risk factors
• Potential reduction in dosage or need for insulin or oral antidiabetic agents
• Enhanced work capacity
• Enriched quality of life and improved sense of well-being

■ In patients treated with insulin or insulin secretagogues, hypoglycemia can be precipitated by exercise and requires a specific plan of monitoring and care to minimize risk.

■ In patients with labile blood glucose levels or microvascular and/or cardiovascular complications, exercise needs to be accompanied by a specific plan of monitoring and care to minimize risk.

PHARMACOLOGIC INTERVENTION

■ When a patient is unable to achieve normal or near-normal glucose levels with dietary changes and exercise, despite adequate education and effort, pharmacologic treatment should be implemented.
• New recommendations suggest that at the diagnosis of type 2 diabetes, in addition to lifestyle intervention, metformin therapy should be initiated concurrently.

■ Pharmacologic intervention is an adjunct to and not a substitute for dietary modification and exercise.

■ The choice among antidiabetic agents should be individualized, taking into account patient preferences, comorbidities/contraindications, goals, ability for self-care management, social support, and finances.

■ Oral antidiabetic agents differ from one another in terms of mechanism of action, physiological effect, pharmacokinetics, and metabolism (Tables 3.8 and 3.9).

■ Insulin secretagogues (sulfonylureas, repaglinide, and nateglinide) stimulate β-cell insulin secretion.

■ The biguanide metformin reduces hepatic glucose overproduction.

■ α-Glucosidase inhibitors delay the absorption of carbohydrates from the intestine.

■ The thiazolidinediones primarily work in fat and muscle to enhance insulin action.

■ Amylinomimetics increase the activity of amylin with effects on glucose and weight.

■ Incretin mimetics increase glucagon-like peptide (GLP)-1 activity with effects on glucose and weight.

■ Dipeptidyl peptidase IV (DPP-4) inhibitors increase the level of incretin hormones.

■ In most patients, a combination of agents is required for adequate glycemic control.

■ Insulin therapy augments the relative insulin deficiency seen in type 2 diabetes. Large doses of insulin may be required because of significant insulin resistance in some patients.

■ Insulin therapy is arguably the most effective and best validated treatment to reduce glucose and risk of complications in diabetes management. It is preferred in the setting of marked (>300 mg/dl) or symptomatic hyperglycemia, in pregnancy, and during hospitalization. It is an appropriate choice for many patients with diabetes.

■ The appropriate insulin regimen depends on the amount of β-cell function remaining, whether oral agents are continued, and the daily glucose pattern as determined by self-monitoring of blood glucose (SMBG), among other factors. Some patients with mild-to-moderate fasting hyperglycemia may be adequately controlled with one injection of intermediate- or long-acting insulin before breakfast or at bedtime. Many patients require a multi-dose regimen consisting of short-acting insulin in combination with either intermediate- or long-acting insulin.

■ Factors that influence the choice of treatments in individual patients are outlined under the topic "Algorithm of Care." When prescribing a pharmacologic treatment, initially a low but effective dose should be used, and the dose should be increased on a schedule suited to that agent until the desired glycemic control is achieved, until the maximum effective dose is reached, or until adverse consequences are observed.

■ Some patients maintained on low doses of medications can discontinue the agents and control glucose levels with nutrition and exercise.

■ From 10 to 20% of patients each year experience loss of glycemic control, which may be due to non-adherence, progression of disease, or the development of a superimposed stressful condition. Control of blood glucose can often be restored after secondary failure of a single agent by addition of a second agent with a different mechanism of action.

■ Each individual antidiabetic therapy is in general well tolerated, but each has relative risks and benefits as well as contraindications. There are inadequate head-to-head studies to establish any one as clearly preferred in all patients.

■ Several drugs in common use today can cause hyperglycemia or hypoglycemia. When possible, these drugs should be avoided.

SPECIAL THERAPEUTIC PROBLEMS

■ Ideally, pregnancy in a patient with diabetes should be planned so that conception occurs when the patient's fasting, preprandial, and postprandial plasma glucose levels are as close to normal as possible. Patients should obtain preconception counseling from the health care team. Referral should be considered if the plasma glucose level is >120 mg/dl (>6.7 mmol/l) or A1C >7% at any time during pregnancy.

■ The major principles governing the management of diabetes during surgery are presented in the section "Special Therapeutic Problems: Diabetes in Hospitalized and Critically Ill Patients." The objectives of management before, during, and after surgery are to optimize healing and minimize risk of perioperative complications by controlling hyperglycemia and avoiding hypoglycemia.

ASSESSMENT OF TREATMENT EFFICACY

■ The therapeutic response to the treatment of diabetes is monitored by determining effects on glucose, blood pressure, lipids, weight, and the signs and symptoms of diabetes complications.

■ Patients can determine the effects of glycemic therapy by SMBG. They can use a daily journal to record food intake, exercise, doses of insulin or oral hypoglycemic agents, symptoms, and results of SMBG. In individuals with type 2 diabetes, the monitoring of urine ketones is usually not necessary.

■ Physicians monitor the responses to treatment by reviewing patients' SMBG results as an index of day-to-day control and with assays for glycated hemoglobin, a reflection of degree of glucose control for the preceding 6–12 weeks.

■ The multiple therapeutic agents and problem-solving using SMBG results should make it possible for most patients to achieve glycemic control goals.

Management

The two major management goals for the patient with type 2 diabetes are to prevent complications and to avoid or alleviate symptoms. Although diabetes is a disease defined on the basis of abnormalities of glucose metabolism, in the setting of type 2 diabetes, it can be argued that aggressive management of blood pressure and lipids, smoking cessation, and anti-platelet therapy are the most important aspects of care. This is because the majority of patients with diabetes succumb to heart attack, stroke, or their consequences. Glucose management is important, since it may have an effect to further reduce cardiovascular risk and clearly lower the risk of development and progression of diabetic retinopathy, nephropathy, and neuropathy. A summary of recommended therapeutic targets for adults with diabetes is provided (Table 3.1).

The evidence that long-term glycemic control can prevent or ameliorate the microvascular and neuropathic complications of diabetes comes from a series of clinical trials. The Diabetes Control and Complications Trial (DCCT) demonstrated the beneficial effects of glycemic control in slowing the progression of retinopathy, nephropathy, and neuropathy in type 1 diabetes. The U.K. Prospective Diabetes Study (UKPDS) demonstrated in patients with new-onset type 2 diabetes that a more intensive use of drug therapy with metformin, sulfonylurea, or insulin in addition to lifestyle intervention caused improved glycemic control and a parallel reduction in the risk of development of combined end points, largely microvascular, with a trend toward reduction in cardiovascular events. In both of these trials, the more intensively treated group exhibited an average A1C of ~7%; thus, an A1C target of <7% has been adopted as the treatment target for patients with diabetes, since the relative risks and benefits at this level of glycemic control are well established.

The absolute risk of end-stage microvascular complications (blindness, dialysis, or amputation) developing over an intermediate time frame (6–10 years) is small at an A1C of 7%, at least in patients with no or early complications. However, there is no threshold or lower limit in A1C below which complications do not develop, thus the rationale for considering lower targets. At levels of A1C lower than 7%, the risk of hypoglycemia increases substantially with each further lowering of A1C, particularly when improvements in control are driven with increasing doses of insulin and sulfonylureas. It is unclear what the absolute benefits and risks are of efforts to achieve A1C targets significantly <7%, and decisions to pursue lower targets must be individualized. The UKPDS and the Steno-2 Study demonstrated

33

Table 3.1 Summary of Recommended Targets for Adults with Diabetes

Glycemic control	A1C <7.0%*
Preprandial plasma glucose	70–130 mg/dl (3.9–7.2 mmol/l)
Postprandial plasma glucose†	<180 mg/dl (<10.0 mmol/l)
Blood pressure	<130/80 mmHg
Lipids‡	
LDL cholesterol	<100 mg/dl (<2.6 mmol/l)
Triglycerides	<150 mg/dl (<1.7 mmol/l)
HDL cholesterol	>40 mg/dl (>1.1 mmol/l)§

Key concepts in setting glycemic goals:

- Goals should be individualized based on duration of diabetes, pregnancy status, age, comorbid conditions, hypoglycemia unawareness, and other individual patient considerations.
- More stringent glycemic goals (i.e., a normal A1C, <6%) may further reduce complications at the cost of increased risk of hypoglycemia (particularly in individuals with type 1 diabetes).
- Postprandial glucose may be targeted if A1C goals are not met, despite reaching preprandial glucose goals.

*Referenced to a nondiabetic range of 4.0–6.0% using a DCCT-based assay.
†Postprandial glucose measurements should be made 1–2 h after the beginning of the meal, generally peak levels in patients with diabetes.
‡Current National Cholesterol Education Program/Adult Treatment Panel III (NCEP/ATP III) guidelines suggest that in patients with triglycerides >200 mg/dl, the "non-HDL cholesterol" (total cholesterol minus HDL) should be used. The goal is <130 mg/dl. Adapted from the ADA and NCEP/ATP III. In individuals with overt cardiovascular disease, a lower LDL cholesterol goal of <70 mg/dl (<1.8 mmol/l), using a high dose of a statin, is an option.
§For women, it has been suggested that the HDL goal be increased by 10 mg/dl. Adapted from the American Diabetes Association, 2008.

that more intensive blood pressure, lipid, and glycemic management resulted in substantial reduction in both microvascular and macrovascular complications. A more specific discussion of cardiovascular risk reduction strategies is given in the chapter "Detection and Treatment of Chronic Complications."

A rational approach to the treatment of elevated blood glucose in patients with type 2 diabetes should include measures that will specifically reverse the underlying pathogenic metabolic disturbances that result in hyperglycemia, i.e., insulin resistance and impaired β-cell function. It is critical to educate patients and their families on self-care practices necessary to manage diabetes. National standards exist for diabetes education programs, and these should be followed. As part of the initial evaluation, a meal plan and exercise program should be developed, pharmacologic therapy should be instituted if necessary, and a monitoring program both at home and in the health care setting needs to be established to assess control. Within this scheme, careful attention to psychosocial influences and/or behavior modification techniques is valuable as outlined in "Strategies for Behavioral Change."

BIBLIOGRAPHY

American Diabetes Association: Standards of medical care in diabetes: 2008 (Position Statement). *Diabetes Care* 31 (Suppl. 1):S12–S54, 2008

Effect of intensive blood-glucose control with metformin on complications in overweight patients with type 2 diabetes (UKPDS 34): UK Prospective Diabetes Study (UKPDS) Group. *Lancet* 352:854–865, 1998

Expert Panel on Detection, Evaluation, and Treatment of High Blood Cholesterol in Adults: Executive Summary of the Third Report of the National Cholesterol Education Program (NCEP) Expert Panel on Detection, Evaluation, and Treatment of High Blood Cholesterol in Adults (Adult Treatment Panel III). *JAMA* 285:2486–2497, 2001

Funnell MM, Brown TL, Childs BP, Haas LB, Hosey GM, Jensen B, Maryniuk M, Peyrot M, Piette JD, Reader D, Siminerio LM, Weinger K, Weiss MA: National standards for diabetes self-management education. *Diabetes Care* 31 (Suppl. 1):S97–S104, 2008

Gaede P, Vedel P, Larsen N, Jensen GV, Parving HH, Pedersen O: Multifactorial intervention and cardiovascular disease in patients with type 2 diabetes. *N Engl J Med* 348:383–393, 2003

Intensive blood-glucose control with sulphonylureas or insulin compared with conventional treatment and risk of complications in patients with type 2 diabetes (UKPDS 33): UK Prospective Diabetes Study (UKPDS) Group. *Lancet* 352:837–853, 1998

Stratton IM, Adler AI, Neil HA, Matthews DR, Manley SE, Cull CA, Hadden D, Turner RC, Holman RR: Association of glycaemia with macrovascular and microvascular complications of type 2 diabetes (UKPDS 35): prospective observational study. *BMJ* 321:405–412, 2000

U.K. Prospective Diabetes Study Group: Tight blood pressure control and risk of macrovascular and microvascular complications in type 2 diabetes: UKPDS 38. *BMJ* 317:703–713, 1998

NUTRITION

Type 2 diabetes develops in most patients because of excessive caloric intake in susceptible individuals. Thus, nutrition therapy is the cornerstone of treatment in type 2 diabetes and should be part of the continuing care of the patient throughout the course of the disease.

Medical nutrition therapy in diabetes is an interactive, collaborative, continuous process of modifying nutrient intake involving the person with diabetes and his or her health care team. It involves:

- Assessment: evaluating an individual's usual food intake, metabolic status, lifestyle, culture, and readiness to make changes
- Goal setting: prioritizing with the patient which areas need improvement and deciding together what is an achievable and realistic goal
- Dietary modification and instruction: teaching the person with diabetes to understand the types and portions of foods to include in a healthy diet, how to read a food label, and the role of carbohydrates in glycemic control so he or she can successfully implement a meal plan that improves metabolic status
- Evaluation of successful implementation and follow-up: self-monitoring of blood glucose (SMBG) may be necessary to evaluate the effects of diet and exercise on glycemic excursions, and routine glycated protein and serum lipid levels provide feedback on macronutrient intake

In some people with mild to moderate diabetes, an appropriate combination of nutrition and exercise is often the only therapeutic intervention needed to effectively control the metabolic abnormalities associated with this disease. The goals of medical nutrition therapy in type 2 diabetes are to:

- Maintain near-normal blood glucose levels
- Normalize serum lipoprotein levels and blood pressure
- Attain and maintain a reasonable body weight
- Promote overall health

Because of the heterogeneous nature of type 2 diabetes, there is no single prescription for dietary modification that will achieve these goals in all patients. The meal plan must be individualized. Diversity in insulin secretion capacity and insulin resistance, as well as personal characteristics related to cultural and social characteristics, lifestyle, age, body weight, and medication regimen, influence strategies to achieve the nutrition goals. Eating habits, attitude, and learning abilities also influence the ability to achieve nutrition goals. Several obstacles to dietary adherence have been identified and should be considered in the dietary assessment and evaluation plan (Table 3.2).

Guidelines for nutritional intervention in individuals with diabetes have been developed that consider the heterogeneity of diabetes (Table 3.3). The success of a particular dietary intervention is evaluated via metabolic parameters, as well as quality of life and body weight. Failure of one intervention strategy may be corrected by using another.

BODY WEIGHT

BMI is used as a practical definition of body weight relative to health risk. It is calculated as weight in kilograms divided by the square of height in meters (kg/m^2).

Table 3.2 Obstacles to Dietary Adherence for Adults with Diabetes

- Resisting temptation: social events, special foods, cues, or cravings trigger unhealthy eating
- Eating out: difficult to control portions and ingredients
- Feeling deprived: regret not being able to eat like people without diabetes
- Negative emotions: attempt to cope by overeating
- Temptation to relapse: feeling of wanting to give up or take a vacation
- Planning/priorities: it takes too much time to prepare foods on the meal plan; other things get in the way
- Family/friends: support is not offered and/or positive behaviors not modeled
- Cost: healthy foods may be more expensive and not easy to obtain

Adapted from Schlundt et al., 1994.

The U.S. Dietary Guidelines for Americans has defined a healthy weight as a BMI of 19–25 kg/m^2. A BMI calculator is available at http://www.cdc.gov/nccdphp/dnpa/bmi/calc-bmi.htm. A BMI >25 kg/m^2 has been generally accepted as a definition of overweight, whereas a BMI >30 kg/m^2 defines obesity. Because body weight profoundly influences insulin resistance, insulin requirements, and subsequent blood glucose control, an appropriate daily caloric intake is integral to the nutrition plan in type 2 diabetes. However, caloric intake may not require modification if BMI is normal or an individual is unwilling or unable to restrict intake.

A weight history is valuable to identify the patient's chronic control of body weight. Although people generally significantly underestimate caloric intake, diet logs, a 24-h diet recall, or a 3-day diet history can be helpful in estimating usual daily caloric intake and eating patterns. This type of assessment will also identify fat, carbohydrate, and protein intake; meal and snack distribution; and micronutrients such as iron, sodium, and calcium.

Normal Weight

Approximately 10–20% of people with type 2 diabetes have a normal BMI and may therefore not need caloric restriction. Asian Americans in particular seem to have a higher risk of diabetes at moderate BMI levels. Because normal-weight individuals have found a way to balance caloric intake with expenditure, the focus of the nutrition plan can be on modifying other components, such as macro- and micronutrients. Carbohydrate content of the diet and the distribution of carbohydrates between meals and snacks becomes the primary intervention.

Carbohydrates have the greatest impact on postprandial blood glucose response. Setting a carbohydrate goal for meals and snacks is one of the best ways to maximize dietary effectiveness. Patients can be taught to increase or decrease carbohydrate intake per meal and/or snack to yield optimal blood glucose results. If they use short-acting insulin, they may be able to adjust insulin dose to compensate for changes in carbohydrate intake by using an insulin-to-carbohydrate ratio. The quality and quantity of fats in the diet can affect lipid levels. Saturated fats, *trans* unsaturated fats, and cholesterol intake may increase circulating atherogenic lipid

Table 3.3 Nutrition Goals, Principles, and Recommendations

Calories

- Sufficient to attain and/or maintain a reasonable body weight for adults, normal growth and development for children and adolescents, and adequate nutrition during pregnancy and lactation
- For weight loss, either low-carbohydrate or low-fat calorie-restricted diets may be effective

Protein

- No more than 0.8 g/kg body wt daily in people with evidence of nephropathy

Fat

- Saturated fat <7% of daily calories
- Intake of *trans* fat should be minimized

Cholesterol

- <200 mg/day

Carbohydrate

- Monitoring carbohydrate intake, whether by carbohydrate counting, exchanges, or experience-based estimation, remains a key strategy in achieving glycemic control
- For individuals with diabetes, the use of the glycemic index and glycemic load may provide a modest additional benefit for glycemic control over that observed when total carbohydrate is considered alone.
- Whole grains and other less processed sources of carbohydrate are preferred

Sweeteners

- Sucrose can be substituted into the meal plan for other sources of carbohydrate; however, care needs to be taken to maintain diet quality and not exceed caloric needs
- Nonnutritive sweeteners approved by the U.S. Food and Drug Administration are safe to consume

Fiber

- 25–35 g/day (14 g fiber per 1,000 kcal)

Sodium

- <2,300 mg/day for hypertensive and normotensive patients

Alcohol

- Moderate usage, i.e., up to two servings of alcohol daily in men and up to one serving daily in women

Vitamins and Minerals

- Same as the general population
- Chromium and vitamins E and C, supplements frequently touted for their benefits in diabetes, do not have proven effectiveness

Goals must always be individualized.

particles, particularly LDL as well as the triglyceride-rich VLDL and remnant particles. Monounsaturated fats often have a beneficial effect on these lipid particles. Intake and proportion of calories from fat should be dictated by the level of dyslipidemia, as well as the level of carbohydrate that optimizes blood glucose.

Diets with varying quantity and sources of carbohydrate, lipids, and proteins have been widely touted in the lay and medical press. Many individuals with type 2 diabetes are presently experimenting with these diets. Since long-term studies have not proven the relative risks and benefits of each, recommending initiation or continuation of these diets should be done on an individual basis, taking into consideration the clinical response and potential for exacerbating dyslipidemia.

Occasionally, particularly in the elderly or in individuals with additional medical problems that increase metabolic needs (such as wound healing), it may be necessary to increase caloric intake. Care should be taken to provide enough calories, protein, vitamins, and minerals to promote healing and anabolic processes.

Overweight

Approximately 80–90% of people with type 2 diabetes are overweight or obese; thus, weight loss is initially the primary treatment goal. Calorie restriction itself may be responsible for improved glucose tolerance, because the loss of as little as 5–10% of body weight improves insulin sensitivity and glucose uptake, reduces insulin secretory requirements, and decreases hepatic glucose production. Weight loss may be most beneficial early in the diagnosis of type 2 diabetes when insulin secretion is most robust, but it clearly continues to have benefits as diabetes progresses.

Weight reduction can be accomplished by a combination of modest caloric restriction, physical activity, behavior modification of eating habits, and psychosocial support. Genetic predisposition to obesity including differences in metabolic and appetite regulation as responses to weight loss may influence a person's ability to lose weight via any regimen. Most individuals will regain lost weight. It has been suggested that such fluctuations in weight are unhealthy for modestly overweight individuals, but little scientific evidence substantiates this concern. On the other hand, the effects of weight gain of as little as 10 kg after age 18 on chronic disease and health are becoming increasingly evident.

Generally, a person's body fat increases with age, although debate exists over the contribution of age-related changes in metabolism versus decreased muscle mass associated with aging. Body fat distributed above the waist increases the risk of developing diabetes, cardiovascular disease (CVD), and hypertension. A waist-to-hip ratio >1.0 or waist ≥40 inches (≥102 cm) in men and waist-to-hip ratio >0.8 or waist ≥35 inches (≥88 cm) in women is associated with increased risk for cardiovascular mortality.

The concept of "dieting" implies a temporary behavior. Obese individuals should be encouraged to make changes they can sustain chronically to attain a reasonable body weight, as determined by BMI. Note that reasonable weight is defined as the weight an individual and health care provider acknowledge as achievable and maintainable, in both the short and long term. This number may not be the same as the defined desirable or ideal BMI (i.e., <25 kg/m^2).

A beneficial weight loss goal is ~2 BMI units or approximately 8–16 lb initially. The U.S. Dietary Guidelines for Americans endorse small weight losses of ½ to

1 lb/week. Not only does an overall weight loss of 5–10 lb improve glucose toler-ance, it also reduces blood pressure and serum lipid levels. Because weight gain in an overweight individual is medically detrimental, and losing weight and keeping it off is extremely difficult, preventing weight gain should be given the same importance as weight loss in an obese individual. A healthy diet plan of moderation combined with daily physical activity is the primary intervention in type 2 diabetes. A 3,500-kcal deficit will produce a loss of 1 lb of body fat. Daily calorie intake should be evaluated with a diet history and adjusted to produce a modest deficit. Generally, a decrease of 500 calories/day is needed to produce a 1-lb loss of fat per week. This can vary, however, based on the individual and his or her willingness to restrict intake and/ or increase activity. Regular exercise enhances weight loss in individuals who also restrict calories and is identified as a predictor for successful weight maintenance.

Alternative approaches for calorie restriction are possible with individuals who are seriously overweight. Very restrictive low-calorie diets (600–800 kcal/day) are sometimes used in type 2 diabetes. This medically supervised approach generally involves a liquid formula, but may be accomplished with high-quality lean protein sources (1.5 g/kg body wt/day) with vitamin and mineral supplementation. Weight loss is rapid (3–5 lb/week), and hyperglycemia generally improves within 24 h of implementation. Near-maximum blood glucose improvement is achieved within 10 days of initiating this regimen. However, this approach should be restricted to individuals who are at least 30% above desirable weight (BMI >30 kg/m²). For some, using this regimen for as short a period as 2–12 weeks can provide the psychological motivation needed to encourage dietary adherence and may in fact improve blood glucose control enough to minimize the need for pharmacologic therapy. Alternat-ing a very-low-calorie dietary regimen with a modest caloric reduction has been used successfully in some studies, as has a weekly "day of fasting," and may be a potential alternative for some individuals. Because a restriction of <1,200 calories for women and <1,500 calories for men is difficult to adhere to and can be nutrition-ally inadequate, most individuals will be more successful if they reduce usual daily intake by 250 calories and increase daily activity by 250 calories. If the diet history is unreliable, approximate daily calorie intake can be estimated by multiplying actual weight in pounds by a factor of 10–15 (the factor decreases with age and decreasing physical activity level).

Pharmacotherapy for the treatment of obesity is considered safe and mod-estly effective when combined with diet and exercise counseling in high-risk obese individuals, including individuals with type 2 diabetes. Each medication has its benefits and risks and should be prescribed only with close medical supervision. Most people will regain the lost weight once the medication is stopped. Therefore, research into the potential long-term use of these drugs is ongoing.

Surgical interventions have been successful in people with a BMI ≥35 kg/m² and in a recent report in type 2 diabetic patients with BMI ≥30 kg/m². A significant and sustained weight loss can be achieved with banding and bypass procedures in most patients but the procedures are costly and can be associated with side effects such as infection, liver disease, dumping syndrome, or even death. The significant amount of weight loss can lead to "remission" of type 2 diabetes, i.e., normaliza-tion of blood glucose without medications, although patients are likely at risk for recurrence of hyperglycemia if they regain weight. Like pharmacotherapy, surgery is only an adjunct to diet and exercise.

People with type 2 diabetes who take insulin secretagogues or insulin may require a decrease or discontinuation of the medication as calorie or carbohydrate restriction is implemented and as weight loss progresses; individuals taking other antihyperglycemic agents may be able to reduce the dosage or number of agents. This reduction may be gradual with a modestly hypocaloric diet or rapid (>50%) with a very-low-calorie diet. In addition, some studies suggest that excessive insulin doses may lead to hunger and overeating, which is counterproductive in obesity.

The results of SMBG may be helpful in making adjustments in nutrition and medication therapy. Frequent follow-up with a dietitian provides problem-solving techniques and encouragement and support for the weight loss efforts (see "Strategies for Behavioral Change"). This follow-up can be done individually or in groups. Appropriate referrals to local hospital programs or other weight loss programs with qualified staff may be useful.

PROTEIN

There is no specific general recommendation for protein intake in type 2 diabetes. Because excessive protein consumption may aggravate glomerular hyperfiltration, the pathophysiological mechanism for the development and progression of renal insufficiency, 0.8–1.0 g/kg body wt/day may represent an optimal goal in those with early nephropathy. Larger amounts are consumed in Western diets (1.2–2.0 g/kg body wt/day). In individuals with more advanced kidney disease, restriction of protein intake to 0.8 g/kg body wt/day may improve measures of renal function including glomerular filtration and urinary albumin excretion. The USDA Food Guide Pyramid recommends 5–7 oz of lean protein daily.

FAT

The proportion of calories derived from carbohydrate and fat depends on food preferences and the desired medical outcome for each individual patient. Lipid abnormalities common in type 2 diabetes are influenced by carbohydrate and fat content of the diet as well as by body weight, genetics, physical activity, and glycemic control. Hypertriglyceridemia and low HDL cholesterol are the most common lipid abnormalities in type 2 diabetes. This dyslipidemia has been shown to be a significant risk factor for CVD in people with and without diabetes.

Low-fat diets, recommended by many experts to reduce LDL cholesterol, may lead some patients to increased carbohydrate intake. Very-high-carbohydrate diets may increase blood glucose and triglyceride levels and lower HDL cholesterol in insulin-resistant patients. However, recent meta-analyses and one large clinical trial suggest that both low-fat and low-carbohydrate diets lower triglycerides (more so for low-carbohydrate diets) and that low-fat diets may be neutral or modestly increase HDL cholesterol (to a lesser extent than low-carbohydrate diets). Low-carbohydrate diets modestly increase LDL cholesterol.

Because saturated fat intake should comprise <7% of total calories, any increase in fat calories should come from monounsaturated fats and polyunsaturated fats. Indeed, studies comparing low-fat with low-carbohydrate diets in type 2 diabetes have used monounsaturated fat in amounts up to 25% of calories. Major sources of monounsaturated fat include olive and canola oils as well as avocado, sesame seeds, and most nuts. Increasing the monounsaturated fat content of the diet without increasing calories can be a challenge that generally requires the assistance of a dietitian. Substituting other vegetable oils for butter, margarine, shortening, and other saturated or high–*trans* fat products can be augmented by adding nuts, olives, and avocado to meals and snacks.

Concern that increasing fat intake could potentially lead to weight gain has proved unfounded. Several controlled clinical studies using high–monounsaturated fat, low-carbohydrate diets did not find excess weight gain. Both short- and intermediate-term weight-loss studies demonstrate that similar or greater weight loss is associated with lower-carbohydrate diet approaches. Reducing fat intake or carbohydrate intake in obese individuals will not necessarily lead to reduced calories; weight loss will occur only if calories are restricted, and approaches to limit fat and particularly highly processed and easily digestible carbohydrates are most appropriate. A low-fat diet without weight loss may or may not result in improved lipid levels in an obese person with type 2 diabetes.

Obese people with diabetes should be given substantial time (weeks to months) on an individualized diet plan that reduces saturated and *trans* fat and less nutrient-dense carbohydrates with a goal of reducing calories. If metabolic parameters such as serum lipids and blood glucose control do not improve, one could consider a moderate-fat increase using monounsaturated fats with a simultaneous further reduction in carbohydrate intake. Close follow-up and monitoring of metabolic parameters should guide further dietary adjustments.

Saturated fats should make up <7–10% of total calories because of their dramatic effect on serum total and LDL cholesterol levels. *Trans* fat should be minimized because it has a similar effect on cholesterol as saturated fats. Currently, adults in the U.S. consume ~13% of total calories from saturated fat. Saturated fatty acids have been shown to be twice as potent in raising plasma cholesterol as polyunsaturated fats are in lowering them. Saturated fatty acids are predominantly found in animal products, but the amount varies between species (Table 3.4). Coconut and palm oils are highly saturated vegetable oils used in baked products, such as cookies and crackers. Whole-milk dairy products and baked goods contribute more to the saturated fat content of the U.S. diet than do meat and meat products. Thus, the most effective way to reduce saturated fat content of the diet is to substitute low-fat milk products, limit meat to lean cuts and reasonable portions, and use baked products made with vegetable oils that have not been hydrogenated. It should be recognized that while epidemiological studies have found a relationship between saturated fat intake and LDL cholesterol levels, there have been no studies that demonstrate reduction in saturated fat intake and improved clinical outcomes.

Cholesterol intake should be limited to <200 mg/day. All animal products, including meat, poultry, eggs, cheese, full-fat dairy products, and shellfish, contain cholesterol. Consuming low-fat dairy products and lean cuts of meat and limiting eggs to ~4/week are the most substantial ways to reduce dietary cholesterol intake. It should be noted that while decreasing cholesterol intake reduces serum cholesterol levels, quantitatively, its effect is less than that of lowering saturated and *trans* fat. The beneficial effect of substituting poultry and fish for red meat is primarily because of the reduced saturated fat content of poultry and fish, since the cholesterol content may be similar. The level of serum cholesterol reduction expected from dietary reduction of fat and cholesterol will vary by individual.

Table 3.4 Fatty Acid Composition of Selected Fats
(Percentage of Total Lipid)

Type of Fat	Monounsaturated Fatty Acid	Polyunsaturated Fatty Acid	Saturated Fatty Acid
Vegetable			
Canola (rapeseed)	66	24	5
Coconut	6	2	87
Corn	25	59	13
Olive	74	8	14
Palm	37	9	49
Peanut	46	32	17
Safflower	12	75	9
Soybean	23	58	14
Animal			
Beef	43	4	40
Butter	29	4	62
Chicken	39	22	28
Lamb	42	7	42
Pork	46	11	36
Salmon	35	29	19
Turkey	32	27	29

Data do not total 100%. Additional components include cholesterol and phytosterols. Adapted from U.S. Department of Agriculture: *Agriculture Handbook No. 8: Composition of Foods.* U.S. Govt. Printing Office, Washington, DC.

Polyunsaturated vegetable fats are liquid at room temperature but can be hydrogenated to yield a more solid product, such as margarine or shortening. In the process, *trans* fatty acids, which are associated with atherogenic lipid profiles, are created. Epidemiological studies have also found an association between the *trans* fatty acid content of the diet and an increased risk of CVD. Vegetable oils and *trans* fat–free margarines are preferred polyunsaturated fat sources.

Fish oil contains polyunsaturated fatty acids in the form of omega-3 fatty acids. Omega-3 fatty acids are converted into ecosinoids and a variety of other derivatives that have been shown to have a beneficial effect on atherogenic lipid profiles, including reduction in serum triglyceride levels. In addition, omega-3 fatty acids increase vascular reactivity, and decreasing platelet aggregation. Because these abnormalities are present in type 2 diabetes, it seems logical that fish oil consumption could be beneficial. Consuming 8 oz of fish each week has been suggested as a safe and effective alternative. All fish contains some fish oil; however, salmon, albacore tuna, mackerel, and herring are the best sources.

CARBOHYDRATE

The amount and type of carbohydrate included in the diet of a person with type 2 diabetes should be individualized and, as with fat and protein, be driven by the predominant metabolic abnormality the patient seeks to improve. If LDL and total cholesterol are elevated, then the initial diet plan should restrict fat to ≤30%. This adjustment would result in ~50–60% of calories being derived from carbohydrate. The clinician should then carefully evaluate daily blood glucose levels and A1C values along with their impact on serum triglycerides and cholesterol to determine if this plan is achieving the desired medical outcomes. If not, a gradual decrease in carbohydrate may be warranted with a subsequent increase in fat, predominantly from monounsaturated fat. The USDA Food Guide Pyramid is a good source for recommending carbohydrate choices for individuals with type 2 diabetes. Its emphasis on whole grains, fruits, and vegetables supplies necessary fiber, vitamins, minerals, and antioxidants to the meal plan. The key is to also teach patients the serving sizes listed from each of the food groups.

Clinical research investigating the impact of carbohydrate-containing foods on blood glucose response has shown that some differences among carbohydrates do exist. Traditionally, starches and grains were thought to produce a lower glycemic response than sugar-containing foods, such as fruits and sweets. Research has not shown this to be true. The longer chains of glucose molecules present in complex carbohydrates, such as starches, do not necessarily yield a flatter blood glucose response curve than the simple carbohydrates found in sugars. Factors such as processing, preparation, and rate of digestion affect the glycemic response of a specific food.

Clinically, the most important determinant of glycemic response to a meal is the total carbohydrate content. Fat and protein contribute little to blood glucose response other than slowing the rate of digestion and absorption of carbohydrate. As a result, once the total amount of carbohydrate to be included in the diet is determined, carbohydrate should be distributed between meals and snacks in a pattern that yields the optimal blood glucose responses. Blood glucose testing is crucial in evaluating carbohydrate distribution. Once the optimal distribution is defined, the therapeutic focus shifts to promoting consistent carbohydrate intake in meals and snacks on a daily basis. Patients requiring insulin can adjust short-acting insulin doses to changing carbohydrate consumption.

Fiber is a nondigestible form of carbohydrate that contributes bulk to the diet and appears to slow down the digestion and absorption of carbohydrate. Soluble fiber, such as that found in oat bran and legumes, can blunt postprandial blood glucose responses and reduce serum cholesterol levels. Insoluble fiber from wheat bran and many fruits and vegetables has little impact on reducing blood glucose or serum cholesterol, but it is necessary for optimal gastrointestinal function. People with diabetes should consume a daily amount of fiber that meets or exceeds the USDA recommendation of 25 g/day (14 g per 1,000 kcal).

Sugar restriction is no longer the primary focus of diet therapy in diabetes. Clinical research has not found sugar-containing foods to be detrimental to blood glucose control when substituted gram for gram for other carbohydrates in the diets of people with diabetes. A modest intake of sugar-containing foods is allowed in the context of a healthy diet. Once again, the USDA Food Guide Pyramid can serve as an excellent guide. Individuals with diabetes can learn to substitute carbohydrate-containing foods using carbohydrate-counting plans or the exchange system. Obese individuals need to be cautioned that high-sugar foods, such as cookies, pastries, and ice creams, are also high in fat and calories. Portion control and understanding how to read food labels are crucial for success.

Although not highly validated by clinical trials, carbohydrate consumption for overweight patients with diabetes should be largely derived from whole grains, vegetables, and fruits, with moderation of the intake of more processed white breads, rice, pasta, cakes, and pastries. The glycemic index is a classification of foods based on their blood glucose–raising potential when studied as single-source meals. Low–glycemic index food raises glucose less after consumption than high–glycemic index foods. The most appropriate use of these concepts is as supplementary to a comprehensive nutrition plan. Some low–glycemic index foods are poor choices for regular consumption in the setting of diabetes because they are high in fat and relatively devoid of other essential nutrients (e.g., chocolate). Some high–glycemic index foods may be good choices for regular consumption, since they are low in calories and full of other nutrients. Finally, in some situations, high–glycemic index foods may be appropriate simply because of convenience (e.g., cereal and skim milk versus a high-fat takeout breakfast sandwich). A recent meta-analysis of low–glycemic index diet trials demonstrated a 0.4% decrement in A1C when compared with high–glycemic index diets.

SUGAR AND FAT SUBSTITUTES

Sorbitol, mannitol, and fructose are commonly used sweeteners that have a lower glycemic effect than either glucose or sucrose (table sugar). Fructose contains the same amount of calories as glucose and sucrose (4 kcal/g); thus, it cannot be used ad libitum, particularly in the hypocaloric diet. In addition, fructose can have a greater effect to raise triglyceride levels than glucose. The sugar alcohols sorbitol and mannitol have only 2–3 kcal/g, but they are often found in products when extra fat has been added. They may cause gastrointestinal distress, such as bloating and diarrhea, when >30 g/day are consumed (10–15 hard candies). Foods containing these sugars must be accounted for in the meal plan. Some sugar alcohols more recently on the market do not have gastrointestinal side effects.

Noncaloric sweeteners such as acesulfame K, aspartame, neotame, saccharin, and sucralose are more than 200 times sweeter than sugar. Their use as tabletop sweeteners and in soft drinks is beneficial in diabetes because they contribute no calories or carbohydrates. However, they may be used in foods that contain other sources of carbohydrates and calories, such as ice cream, cookies, and puddings. These foods need to be worked into the meal plan appropriately.

Fat substitutes currently on the market are derived primarily from carbohydrate or protein, reducing their caloric value from 9 to 4 kcal/g. However, the use of fat substitutes in foods such as yogurt, ice cream, and salad dressings increases the carbohydrate content of the products above their usual level. Individuals should be advised to consider the carbohydrate level when using such foods.

Newer fat substitutes, such as olestra, are fat replacers made from fat that have been modified to be totally nondigestible and therefore not absorbed. As a result, olestra adds no fat or fat calories to products. It can also produce gastrointestinal distress and occasionally is associated with deficiencies in fat-soluble vitamins. Sugar- and fat-modified foods may be beneficial to people with diabetes by helping them reduce their fat, carbohydrate, and calorie intake. However, they are not necessary to follow a healthy diet and should only be suggested as alternatives.

VITAMINS AND MINERALS

Some studies have suggested that patients with diabetes have a high prevalence of subclinical micronutrient deficiency. Limited randomized controlled trials have demonstrated modest benefits of multivitamin/mineral supplementation among patients with type 2 diabetes, particularly among elderly adults on calorie-restricted diets. However, there is currently no evidence for an increased need for vitamins or minerals in diabetes above the current recommended daily allowance. Although a role for the use of antioxidants, such as β-carotene, vitamin E, and vitamin C, has been hypothesized in diabetes, clinical trials have not demonstrated benefits and in some cases have suggested risks.

Chromium and its role in preventing and treating type 2 diabetes are still controversial. Chromium potentiates insulin action, and a deficiency of chromium has been implicated in causing insulin resistance characterized by elevated blood glucose levels, triglycerides, and reduced HDL. Whole-grain products, nuts and seeds, and protein-rich foods are the best sources of chromium, but these can realistically provide only ~50 µg/day. Studies with chromium supplementations have been mixed in their results. Therefore, chromium supplementation is not currently recommended.

A combination of folic acid (1 mg), vitamin B12 (400 µg), and pyridoxine (10 mg) has been shown to reduce homocysteine. Elevated homocysteine has been associated with cardiovascular risk in various epidemiological studies. However, such vitamin combinations have not been demonstrated to reduce CVD events in large-scale clinical trials and therefore are not recommended in diabetes care.

Sodium recommendations for people with diabetes are no more restrictive than for the general population. Most health authorities recommend no more than 2,400 mg/day of sodium for the general population. For people with diabetes, with or without hypertension, <2,300 mg/day of sodium is recommended.

ALCOHOL

Strict abstinence from alcohol is not necessary for patients with diabetes. In most cases, moderate amounts of alcohol (up to two servings daily for men and one serving daily for nonpregnant women, as recommended for the general population) are allowable in diabetes. Recent studies in the general population have shown reduced CVD mortality to be associated with moderate alcohol consumption. Nevertheless, the observational data are insufficient to support routinely recommending alcohol intake in people with diabetes. Obviously, alcohol consumption is not recommended for people with conditions such as pregnancy, alcoholism, cirrhosis of the liver, and symptomatic neuropathy.

Before a patient may include alcohol in his or her eating plan, the potential problems associated with alcohol consumption should be considered, e.g., alcohol consumption by a person who is fasting (>5 h) or undernourished may lead to hypoglycemia. This can be a serious problem in patients taking insulin or an oral hypoglycemic agent who skip meals. A patient's ability to follow the prescribed management plan will be impaired if he or she is intoxicated. Additionally, alcohol ingestion may be associated with significant elevations in fasting and postprandial plasma triglyceride levels in people with hypertriglyceridemia. Alcohol should be consumed with food, especially for individuals on insulin.

BIBLIOGRAPHY

American Diabetes Association: Nutrition recommendations and interventions for diabetes (Position Statement). *Diabetes Care* 31 (Suppl. 1):S61–S78, 2008

Barringer TA, Kirk JK, Santaniello AC, Foley KL, Michielutte R: Effect of a multivitamin and mineral supplement on infection and quality of life: a randomized, double-blind, placebo-controlled trial. *Ann Intern Med* 138:365–371, 2003

Brand-Miller J, Hayne S, Petocz P, Colagiuri S: Low–glycemic index diets in the management of diabetes: a meta-analysis of randomized controlled trials. *Diabetes Care* 26:2261–2267, 2003

DCCT Research Group: Expanded role of the dietitian in the Diabetes Control and Complications Trial: implications for clinical practice. *J Am Diet Assoc* 93:758–764, 1993

Dixon JB, O'Brien PE, Playfair J, Chapman L, Schachter LM, Skinner S, Proietto J, Bailey M, Anderson M: Adjustable gastric banding and conventional therapy for type 2 diabetes: a randomized controlled trial. *JAMA* 299:316–323, 2008

Look-AHEAD Research Group: Reduction in weight and cardiovascular risk factors in individuals with type 2 diabetes: one year results of the Look-AHEAD trial. *Diabetes Care* 30:1374–1383, 2007

Mooradian AD, Failla M, Hoogwerf B, Maryniuk M, Wylie-Rosett J: Selected vitamins and minerals in diabetes. *Diabetes Care* 17:464–479, 1994

Nordmann AJ, Nordmann A, Briel M, Keller U, Yancy WS Jr, Brehm BJ, Bucher HC: Effect of low-carbohydrate vs. low-fat diets on weight loss and cardiovascular risk factors: a meta-analysis of randomized controlled trials. *Arch Intern Med* 166:285–293, 2006

Schlundt DG, Rea MR, Kline SS, Pichert JW: Situational obstacles to dietary adherence for adults with diabetes. *JAMA* 94:874–876, 1994

U.S. Department of Agriculture: *The Food Guide Pyramid.* Hyattsville, MD, Human Nutrition Information Service, 1992

Yeh GY, Eisenberg DM, Kaptchuk TJ, Phillips RS: Systematic review of herbs and dietary supplements for glycemic control in diabetes. *Diabetes Care* 26:1277–1294, 2003

EXERCISE

Exercise in type 2 diabetes can be a useful therapeutic tool. To be effective, an exercise regimen requires individualization and monitoring. Specific precautions need to be taken in some individuals to ensure benefit and minimize risk.

Both obesity and inactivity contribute to the development of glucose intolerance in the person genetically predisposed to diabetes. Regular exercise may delay or prevent type 2 diabetes onset in high-risk populations.

POTENTIAL BENEFITS OF EXERCISE

Regular exercise in type 2 diabetes has the potential to:

- Reduce cardiovascular risk factors such as hyperlipidemia and hypertension
- Augment weight-reduction diets
- Improve blood glucose control by enhancing insulin sensitivity
- Reduce dosage or need for insulin or oral medications
- Enhance quality of life
- Improve psychological well-being

Improved Insulin Sensitivity/Glucose Tolerance

Insulin resistance is a feature of type 2 diabetes. Exercise enhances insulin sensitivity and increases skeletal muscle glucose uptake, both during and for 48 h after the activity. Thus, repeated bouts of exercise at regular intervals are most beneficial to reduce the glucose intolerance associated with type 2 diabetes. This exercise-induced enhanced sensitivity to insulin occurs without changes in body weight. Unless contraindicated by other health problems, exercise should be a component of the treatment regimen in all people with type 2 diabetes, regardless of whether there is a need for weight reduction.

Exercise may result in enhanced effects of insulin or oral secretagogues. Therefore, careful SMBG is required to minimize hypoglycemia.

Exercise and Weight Reduction

Physical activity is recognized as an important part of weight-reduction programs. Although exercise, in absence of caloric restriction, is inconsistent in promoting weight loss, exercise has been consistently identified as the strongest predictor for long-term maintenance of lost weight. Exercise increases energy expenditure to create a greater caloric deficit than a hypocaloric diet alone. Exercise also increases lean body mass (muscle tissue), which helps to maintain the metabolic rate that otherwise declines with loss of body weight. Of particular importance is the fact that aerobic exercise decreases abdominal (central) adiposity. Because central obesity increases cardiovascular risk, this finding is relevant for patients with type 2 diabetes.

Cardiovascular Conditioning

The value of physical training in ameliorating risk factors for CVD has been amply demonstrated in nondiabetic individuals. Exercise is associated with a reduction in circulating levels of VLDL and LDL cholesterol and triglycerides and increases in levels of HDL cholesterol. Furthermore, exercise is associated with decreases in blood pressure and heart rate, both at rest and during exercise, as well as increases in maximum oxygen uptake and total working capacity.

The beneficial effects of exercise on risk factors in patients with type 2 diabetes have not been studied extensively, but it is reasonable to assume that exercise may help to prevent or slow cardiovascular complications in this particularly susceptible group of individuals. Again, however, the cardiovascular and metabolic benefits of exercise are sustained only as the result of the sum of effects of individual sessions of exercise or as a result of long-term changes in body composition.

Psychological Benefits

Exercise training and fitness are often associated with decreased anxiety, improved mood and self-esteem, and an increased sense of well-being. Enhanced quality of life may be a secondary benefit to strength training (increased muscle mass, flexibility, and range of motion), particularly in the aging population in which type 2 diabetes predominates. Regular exercise may improve glucose control in part by providing a coping mechanism for stress.

PRECAUTIONS AND CONSIDERATIONS

Exercise of any kind is safe for most people with type 2 diabetes. However, special precautions should be taken. Because many individuals with type 2 diabetes have led sedentary lives for years, they are frequently deconditioned. The role of stress testing before beginning an exercise program is controversial. There is no evidence that such testing is routinely necessary for individuals planning moderate-intensity activity such as walking. Perhaps it should be considered in previously sedentary individuals at moderate to high risk of CVD who want to undertake vigorous exercise programs.

The medical evaluation should include the following:

- Determination of glycemic control
- Cardiovascular examination (blood pressure, peripheral pulses, bruits)
- Neurological examination
- Dilated fundoscopic examination, especially if proliferative retinopathy is present or suspected

Because most people with type 2 diabetes have had the disease for several years before diagnosis, newly diagnosed patients should be examined for hypertension, neuropathy, retinopathy, and nephropathy (Table 3.5). Silent ischemic heart disease can be present without chest pain. Autonomic neuropathy and β-blockers may interfere with maximal heart rate and exercise performance. This is in addition to the already observed 15–20% lower age-matched maximal heart rate found in people with type 2 diabetes. Lower target heart rates and less stressful exercise regimens

Table 3.5 Precautions for Patients with Medical Complications

- Insensitive feet or peripheral vascular insufficiency
  - Avoid running
  - Choose walking, cycling, or swimming
  - Emphasize proper footwear and daily foot inspection
- Untreated or recently treated proliferative retinopathy: avoid exercises associated with:
  - Increased intra-abdominal pressure
  - Valsalva-like maneuvers
  - Rapid head movements
  - Eye trauma
- Hypertension
  - Avoid heavy lifting
  - Avoid Valsalva-like maneuvers
  - Choose exercises that primarily involve the lower-extremity rather than upper-extremity muscle groups

are recommended in these individuals. Strenuous exercise is contraindicated for patients with poor metabolic control and for those with significant diabetic complications (particularly active proliferative retinopathy, significant CVD, and neuropathy).

Foot sensitivity and adequacy of circulation should be evaluated, and patients with impairment should avoid forms of exercise that involve trauma to the feet. Proper footwear is important.

Most patients with active proliferative retinopathy and/or hypertension should avoid strenuous, high-intensity exercises associated with Valsalva-like maneuvers (e.g., weight lifting and certain types of isometrics). High-intensity anaerobic activities such as weight lifting involving near-maximal effort and small numbers of repetition can increase glucose. Rhythmic exercises involving the lower extremities (e.g., walking, jogging, swimming, and cycling) can potentiate the hypoglycemic effects of both oral medications and insulin. Hypoglycemia can occur during or as much as 12–24 h after the exercise session. Blood glucose monitoring is beneficial in guiding medication adjustments to prevent exercise-induced hypoglycemia. Insulin may need to be decreased on days during which exercise is performed (Table 3.6). This is particularly important if exercise is an adjunct to weight loss. It would be counterproductive to repeatedly have to treat a hypoglycemic reaction with food or to consume extra food to prevent hypoglycemia in patients on a hypocaloric diet.

Special precautions should be taken when a patient requires or uses drugs that may make him or her more susceptible to exercise-induced hypoglycemia. For example, alcohol and very high doses of salicylates should be avoided because they may themselves produce hypoglycemia. The β-adrenergic blocking agents may prevent the rapid hepatic glyconeolytic responses that normally correct hypoglycemia as well as mask adrenergic symptoms of hypoglycemia. Certain other drugs may potentiate the action of sulfonylureas.

Table 3.6 Guidelines for Safe Exercise

- At all times, patients should carry an identification card and wear a bracelet, necklace, or tag that identifies them as having diabetes.
- If the patient uses insulin:
  - Avoid exercise during peak insulin action
  - Administer insulin away from working limbs
- If the patient takes a single daily dose of intermediate-acting insulin, decrease the dose before exercise by as much as 30–35%.
- If the patient uses a combination of short- and intermediate-acting insulin, decrease or omit the short-acting insulin dose and decrease the dose of intermediate-acting insulin by up to one-third on days when exercise is planned. This may produce hyperglycemia later in the day that requires a second injection of short-acting insulin.
- If the patient uses only short-acting insulin, reduce the pre-exercise dose and reduce the post-exercise dose based on SMBG. The total dose may need to be reduced by as much as 30–50% on days when exercise is planned.
- Be alert for signs of hypoglycemia during and for several hours after exercise. Have immediate access to a source of readily absorbable carbohydrate (such as glucose tablets) to treat hypoglycemia.
- Take sufficient fluids before, after, and, if necessary, during exercise to prevent dehydration.

Patients with type 2 diabetes controlled by diet alone or medications that do not cause hypoglycemia can perform exercise in the same manner as people without diabetes. Supplementary food before, during, or after activity is unnecessary, because hypoglycemia is not a risk.

THE EXERCISE PRESCRIPTION

The key to a successful exercise program is individualization: it must take into account the interests, initial physical condition, and motivation of the patient. A safe exercise prescription requires a complete medical evaluation and specific instructions for managing the exercise program. The patient should start slowly, exercise at regular intervals at least three to four times per week, and gradually increase the duration, intensity, and frequency of the exercise. The Institute of Medicine recommends 1 h daily of a moderately vigorous program.

Timing the exercise session in type 2 diabetes may be used advantageously. It appears that exercise performed after 4:00 p.m. may reduce hepatic glucose output and decrease fasting glycemia. Exercise after eating may reduce the postprandial hyperglycemia commonly observed in type 2 diabetes. Because exercise is so important, it should be encouraged regardless of when it is performed.

Activity

The type of exercise a patient chooses should be tailored to his or her physical capacity and interests. Most patients can, at a minimum, undertake a walking program safely. Aerobic activities, such as biking, swimming, jogging, and dancing, should be encouraged as well. Biking and swimming are particularly valuable in patients with neuropathy, where foot placement and steady gait may be compromised.

A complete exercise program also includes muscle-strengthening exercises, such as lifting light weights three times a week, targeting all major muscle groups, progressing to three sets of 8–10 repetitions at a weight that cannot be lifted more than 8–10 times. At least initial supervision and periodic assessment by a qualified exercise specialist is recommended to optimize benefits and minimize risks of resistance training.

Armchair exercises can be performed by individuals who are confined to a chair or who may have limited mobility. Flexibility stretches are useful during warm-up and cool-down periods. These not only prepare muscles for an aerobic workout, but also promote improved range of motion, which is especially valuable in elderly people.

Intensity

There are several ways to monitor exercise intensity. One recommendation is to sustain a heart rate at ~60–80% of the maximal heart rate. Generating even 50% of maximum heart rate may be beneficial. Previously sedentary patients should never be given a high-end heart rate goal unless an exercise stress test is performed. However, a low-end heart rate goal (i.e., <110 beats/min) can be given without stress testing.

Another alternative is to use a rating of perceived exertion. Patients can be guided to work hard, generally at a brisk pace where a light sweat may be present and they perceive they are working. At this pace, they should have enough breath to carry on a conversation. In general, patients should not focus primarily on the intensity of activity, because any activity is preferred to a sedentary lifestyle.

Duration and Frequency

To improve glycemic control, assist with weight maintenance, and reduce risk of CVD, at least 150 min/week of moderate-intensity aerobic physical activity (50–70% of maximum heart rate) and/or at least 90 min/week of vigorous aerobic exercise (>70% of maximum heart rate) are recommended. The physical activity should be distributed over at least 3 days/week and with no more than 2 consecutive days without physical activity. Greater CVD risk reduction is expected with ≥4 h/week of moderate to vigorous aerobic and/or resistance exercise. For long-term maintenance of major weight loss (>13.6 kg/30 lb), even larger volumes of exercise (7 h/week of moderate or vigorous aerobic physical activity) may be helpful.

BIBLIOGRAPHY

American Diabetes Association: Standards of medical care in diabetes: 2008 (Position Statement). *Diabetes Care* 31 (Suppl. 1):S12–S54, 2008

American Diabetes Association: Physical activity/exercise and type 2 diabetes (Position Statement). *Diabetes Care* 29:1433–1439, 2006

Ruderman N, Devlin JT, Schneider SH, Krisra A (Eds.): *Handbook of Exercise in Diabetes.* Alexandria, VA, American Diabetes Association, 2002

Haskell WL, Lee IM, Pate RR, Powell KE, Blair SN, Franklin BA, Macera CA, Heath GW, Thompson PD, Bauman A, American College of Sports Medicine, American Heart Association: Physical activity and public health: updated recommendation for adults from the American College of Sports Medicine and the American Heart Association. *Circulation* 116:1081–1093, 2007

PHARMACOLOGIC INTERVENTION

Since 1995, the pharmacotherapy of type 2 diabetes has been revolutionized with seven new classes of antihyperglycemic therapies as well as improvements in sulfonylureas and insulins. Also, recent publications and newer agents have set the stage for starting pharmacotherapy earlier, when glucose levels are only modestly elevated.

First, the UKPDS demonstrated that patients with an average A1C of 7% treated with insulin, metformin, or sulfonylurea (if their fasting glucose was >108 mg/dl) were associated with improved outcomes when compared with patients continuing diet and exercise until symptoms of hyperglycemia developed. Second, the new emphasis on screening for diabetes coupled with the new definition of diabetes (fasting plasma glucose [FPG] ≥126 mg/dl [≥7 mmol/l]) has focused attention on less severely affected people who have previously not been identified or treated. Third, many of the new oral agents do not cause hypoglycemia when used alone, making early and more intensive treatment safer.

AVAILABLE AGENTS

The agents now available for treating type 2 diabetes are listed in Table 3.7. They may be divided into three categories: those enhancing the effectiveness of insulin, those increasing the supply of insulin, and those working in non-insulin hormonal systems. Metformin, α-glucosidase inhibitors, and thiazolidinediones enhance the effectiveness of injected or endogenous insulin. They have principal actions at the liver, in the intestinal lumen, and in muscle and adipose tissue, respectively, all assisting whatever insulin is available in regulating glucose levels.

Sulfonylureas and the non-sulfonylurea secretagogues repaglinide and nateglinide as well as injected insulins increase the circulating levels of insulin. Sulfonylureas, repaglinide, and nateglinide increase the secretion of insulin into the portal circulation, whereas injected insulin supplements endogenously produced insulin levels in the systemic circulation.

The other hormonal systems that can now be pharmacologically modulated to lower glucose include amylin and the incretin hormone glucagon-like peptide 1 (GLP-1). These hormones variously affect glucagon and insulin secretion, gastric emptying, and appetite.

Because the mechanisms of action of all these classes of agents differ, except perhaps in the case of sulfonylureas and the non-sulfonylurea secretagogues, they demonstrate complementary or additive effects in most cases. Some features of these drugs are shown in Table 3.8.

Agents Enhancing the Effectiveness of Insulin

Because these agents are unlikely to cause hypoglycemia and can be used very early in the natural history of type 2 diabetes, they will be discussed first.

Metformin. Metformin belongs to the biguanide class of drugs. After administration, the highest concentrations of metformin are found in the gut and liver. It is not metabolized, but is rapidly cleared from plasma by the kidney. Because of rapid clearance, metformin is usually taken two to three times daily or in an

Table 3.7 Agents Available in the U.S.

Class	Agent Generic Name	Brand Name
Enhance the Effects of Insulin		
Biguanide	Metformin	Glucophage
Thiazolidinedione or "glitazones"	Rosiglitazone Pioglitazone	Avandia Actos
α-Glucosidase inhibitor	Acarbose Miglitol	Precose Glyset
Augment the Supply of Insulin		
Sulfonylurea	Tolbutamide Chlorpropamide Tolazamide Glipizide, Glipizide ER Glyburide Glimepiride	Orinase Diabinese Tolinase Glucotrol, Glucotrol XL DiaBeta, Micronase, Glynase Amaryl
Non-sulfonylurea or "glinide"	Repaglinide Nateglinide	Prandin Starlix
Modify Non-Insulin Hormonal Systems		
Amylinomimetic	Pramlintide	Symlin
Incretin mimetic	Exenatide	Byetta
Dipeptidyl peptidase IV inhibitor	Sitagliptin	Januvia

extended release formulation once or twice daily. Its mechanism of action is not completely understood; recent studies suggest that it activates AMP-activated protein kinase, an intracellular signal of depleted cellular energy stores. Its primary pharmacologic effect is reducing elevated hepatic glucose production without impairing the ability of the patient to respond to fasting by increasing hepatic glucose production. It also may improve the response of muscle to insulin (especially at higher dosages), perhaps by reducing calorie intake or by alleviating "glucose toxicity" in muscles by lowering plasma glucose levels. Treatment with full dosage typically reduces A1C by 1–2%. When metformin is started, weight does not increase or declines slightly, and lipid profiles and blood pressure may improve minimally as well.

The main concern regarding metformin treatment historically has been lactic acidosis. However, recent experience suggests that fatal lactic acidosis associated with metformin is extremely rare. To minimize this risk, metformin should not be given to patients with significant renal disease (serum creatinine >1.4 for women or >1.5 for men), or to those with serious hepatic or cardiovascular decompensation, and should be used with caution in the elderly. It is worth noting that renal function is related to serum creatinine only loosely and that the relationship is influenced

Table 3.8 Comparisons of Therapies for Type 2 Diabetes

Property	Lifestyle Modification	Insulins	Sulfonylureas	Metformin
Target tissue	Muscle or fat	β-Cell supplement	β–Cell	Liver
△ A1C (monotherapy)	Variable	1–2%	1–2%	1–2%
Fasting effect	Good	Excellent	Good	Good
Postprandial effect	Good	Excellent	Good	Good
Severe hypoglycemia	No	Yes	Yes	No
Dosing interval	Continuous	q.d. to continuous	q.d. to t.i.d.	b.i.d. or t.i.d.
△ Weight (lb/yr)	+1	+3	+1–3	0 to –6
△ Insulin	Variable	Increase	Increase	Modest decrease
△ LDL	Minimal decrease	Minimal decrease	None	Decrease
△ HDL	Minimal increase	None	None	Increase
△ TG	Minimal decrease	Decrease	None	Decrease
Common problem	Recidivism, injury	Hypoglycemia, weight gain	Hypoglycemia, weight gain	Transient GI symptoms
Rare problem				Lactic acidosis
Contraindications	None	None	Allergy	Renal failure Liver failure CHF >80 yr old
Cost ($/mo)	0–200	30–450	10–15	30–60
Maximum effective dose		1–2 units/kg/day	½ max or double starting	1000 mg b.i.d.

HDL, high-density lipoprotein; LDL, low-density lipoprotein; max, maximum; Mod, moderate; N, nateglinide; P, pioglitazone; Re, repaglinide; Ro, rosiglitazone; TG, triglycerides.

by weight, age, and creatinine production. Because of these issues, it is recommended that in individuals >80 years of age, renal function should be measured using a 24-h urine collection before prescribing metformin. In other patients, it may be worthwhile estimating glomerular filtration rate (GFR) by using the MDRD equation, available online at http://www.nephron.com/mdrd/default.html. For normal renal function or stage 1 and 2 chronic kidney disease (>60 ml/min/1.73 m^2), full doses of metformin are reasonable. For patients with stage 3 chronic kidney disease (30–59 ml/min/1.73 m^2), half-maximal doses of metformin are arguably reasonable. For patients with stage 4 and 5 kidney disease (GFR <30 ml/min/1.73 m^2), metformin should be avoided.

Substantial enthusiasm about the use of metformin as the drug of choice in the treatment of diabetes is expressed in most guidelines as a result of its superior performance in overweight patients in the UKPDS. In that subgroup, initial treatment with metformin as opposed to sulfonylureas and insulin was associated

	α-Glucosidase Inhibitors	Glitazones	Meglitinides	Exenatide	Pramlintide	Sitagliptin
	Gut	Muscle	Beta cell	Various	Brain	Various
	0.5–1%	0.5–2%	Re: 1–2% N: 0.5–1%	~1%	~0.5%	~0.8%
	Poor	Good	Re: Mod N: Poor	Poor	Poor	Good
	Excellent	Good	Re: Good N: Exc	Excellent	Excellent	Good
	No	No	Re: Yes N: No	No	No	No
	b.i.d. to q.i.d.	P: q.d. Ro: q.d. or b.i.d.	t.i.d. to q.i.d. with meals	b.i.d.	t.i.d.	q.d.
	0 to −10	+1–13	+1–3	−6 to −12	−3 to −6	+1
	Modest decrease	Decrease	Increase	Increase	None	Increase
	Minimal decrease	Increase	None	None	None	None
	None	Increase	None	Decrease	None	None
	Minimal decrease	P: Decrease Ro: None	None	Decrease	None	Decrease
	Flatulence	Weight gain, edema, anemia	Hypoglycemia	GI	GI	None
		Hepatotoxicity?				Stevens-Johnson
	Intestinal disease	Hepatocellular disease		None	None	Dose reduce in renal failure
	40–80	75–180	70–110	170–200	200–400	171
	50 mg t.i.d.	P: 45 mg q.d. Ro: 4 mg b.i.d.	Re: 2 mg t.i.d. N: 120 mg t.i.d.	10 y b.i.d.	120 y ac	100 mg q.d.

with less hypoglycemia and weight gain and a statistically significant reduction in all-cause mortality. Metformin has been associated with modest beneficial changes in lipids, blood pressure, weight, and other cardiovascular risk markers associated with insulin resistance in some but not all studies.

Metformin should be started at a low dose and titrated upward slowly. The starting dose of metformin is 500 mg once or twice daily with breakfast and/or the evening meal. After 1–2 weeks, the dose may be increased sequentially until unacceptable adverse effects arise or the patient is taking an adequate or the maximally effective dose of 1,000 mg b.i.d. Metformin's main side effects are gastrointestinal, notably anorexia, nausea, or diarrhea. These side effects are frequent (10–30%) at dosages above 1,750 mg daily, but may occur and persist at lower doses in ~5% of patients. In many patients, these side effects are transient and can be minimized by slow titration of the dose and can be alleviated by dose reduction when persistent. Metformin is generally better tolerated when taken with a meal. For patients who experience significant nausea with metformin, sometimes extended release formulations will be better tolerated. Because metformin is well tolerated, it is reasonable to use the maximal dose of metformin in nearly all individuals.

Thiazolidinediones/glitazones. The thiazolidinediones, more commonly referred to as glitazones, bind to peroxisome proliferator–activated receptor (PPAR)-γ, a type of nuclear regulatory protein, altering the transcription of numerous genes believed to be important in fat and glucose metabolism. The metabolic effects of these agents develop gradually over several weeks and may take 3–6 months to reach full expression. The major site of action seems to be in adipose tissue, enhancing the expression of genes responsible for triglyceride storage. Glitazones may also initiate the development of new fat cells from stromal precursors, particularly in the subcutaneous compartment. The increase in the ability to store triglyceride results in a reduction in serum free fatty acid concentrations and a net shift of fat from other tissues such as muscle, liver, and β-cells, resulting in an improvement in insulin action and insulin secretion. The glitazones can also alter the expression of a number of adipokines, which also may result in improvement in insulin action (see "Pathogenesis").

Troglitazone was the first thiazolidinedione approved for clinical use in the U.S.; however, it was withdrawn from the market as a result of rare cases of severe hepatotoxicity. The remaining agents, rosiglitazone and pioglitazone, appear not to be associated with hepatotoxicity. Nevertheless, it is suggested that these agents not be used in patients with active liver disease or in patients with transaminases elevated >2.5-fold over the upper limits of normal. Intermittent liver function test monitoring should be performed in patients treated with glitazones.

The glitazones are associated with reductions of A1C on the order of 1–2%, reducing both fasting and postprandial glucose substantially. Because of their insulin-sensitizing nature, they are associated with a reduction in glucose with either no change or a reduction in insulin levels. These agents also have effects on β-cell function and are associated with a normalization of the proinsulin-to-insulin ratio, improved β-cell secretory dynamics, and reactivity. In the ADOPT (A Diabetes Outcome Progression Trial) study, rosiglitazone was associated with a lower risk of secondary failure of glycemic control than metformin and particularly glyburide. Treatment with glitazones may also slow the rate of decline of β-cell function observed in patients treated with sulfonylurea or metformin.

Fluid retention and weight gain have been the main adverse events in human trials of glitazones. The weight gain is least when the glitazones are used in combination with diet and exercise or with metformin (generally a few pounds over the first year versus placebo) and greater when these agents are used in combination with insulin or sulfonylureas (average weight gain on the order of 5–10 lb over the first year). The fluid retention most commonly results in edema. Cases of congestive heart failure have been precipitated by glitazone treatment, but these are more often characterized by peripheral edema and not by pulmonary edema and do not seem to be associated with increased mortality. Although some patients with congestive heart failure that develops during glitazone therapy have an echocardiographic picture of systolic dysfunction, most have diastolic dysfunction and as such were unrecognized premorbidly. There is no evidence in humans that there is an untoward effect of glitazones on cardiac performance. Because of the higher risk of fluid retention, it is recommended that, in patients treated with insulin with peripheral edema or with a history of cardiac disease, glitazone treatment should be initiated with the lowest dose and titrated slowly over months while monitoring therapeutic response and potential side effects. Patients should be educated regarding the possibility of fluid retention presenting as edema, dyspnea, or fatigue and should be counseled to return for evaluation should these problems develop. Diuretics seem effective to minimize symptomatology; in one study, thiazide diuretic and spironolactone was more effective than furosemide. There is anecdotal evidence that the risk of fluid retention is higher in patients treated with non-steroidal anti-inflammatory drugs and calcium-channel blockers and perhaps less in patients treated with angiotensin-converting enzyme inhibitors, angiotensin receptor blockers, and diuretics, but this has not been systematically studied in clinical trials. The glitazones are contraindicated in patients with class III and class IV heart failure because of these concerns and the lack of studies to evaluate their safety and efficacy in those populations.

A more recently recognized adverse event associated with glitazone therapy is bone fractures in postmenopausal women. It has not been conclusively demonstrated that this is related to bone demineralization, and intriguingly the fractures have been in distal extremities (hands and feet) and not in more classic osteoporotic fracture sites such as the hip and spine. Small studies have demonstrated increases in markers of bone turnover after the institution of glitazone therapy.

The glitazones also seem to have variable effects on circulating lipids. Rosiglitazone is associated with an elevation in serum HDL cholesterol and LDL particle size with a moderate increase of apolipoprotein (Apo)B and LDL particle number. Pioglitazone is associated with improvements in serum HDL cholesterol, triglycerides, LDL particle size, LDL particle number, and ApoB. Both agents demonstrate moderate effects on a number of inflammatory and cellular markers associated with excess cardiovascular risk. The PROactive trial is the only completed clinical trial to examine CVD events with glitazones; it was a randomized, double-blind, placebo-controlled study in over 5,000 patients with type 2 diabetes and clinical CVD. Subjects were randomized to placebo or to 45 mg/day pioglitazone and otherwise treated according to guidelines for hyperglycemia and major cardiovascular risk factors. The primary end point was the time from randomization to a broad set of macrovascular end points. Pioglitazone was associated with a 10% reduction in the primary end point, which was not statistically significant. However, for the "principal" secondary end point, time from randomization to death, nonfatal MI (excluding silent MI), and stroke, pioglitazone therapy was associated with a 16% reduction, which was marginally statistically significant but could largely be accounted for by improvements in glycemia, lipids, and blood pressure compared with placebo. The benefits were in part mitigated by an increased incidence of heart failure, weight gain, and edema. Recent meta-analyses suggested that rosiglitazone may be associated with an increase in adverse cardiovascular end points, particularly nonfatal myocardial infarction; this has resulted in additional warnings in the prescribing information for rosiglitazone.

The glitazones should be started at the lowest dose, with follow-up generally in 4–12 weeks. It will generally take 2–4 weeks to see much of a response in self-monitored blood glucose and 3–6 months to see the full A1C benefit. The maximal dose seems to be associated with modest additional glucose-lowering effect, particularly in combination therapy, but with a greater proclivity for weight gain and other adverse events.

α-Glucosidase inhibitors. Acarbose and miglitol are α-glucosidase inhibitors; they work in the intestinal lumen, where they competitively inhibit enzymes that hydrolyze polysaccharides into simple sugars. Their main effect is on the metabolism of starches, but cleavage of the disaccharide sucrose to glucose and fructose is also reduced. Cleavage of lactose is unaffected. The result of this action is to delay absorption of dietary carbohydrates until they have passed to the mid or distal small bowel, resulting in reduced postprandial peaks of plasma glucose. They have little effect on fasting glucose. To achieve their glucose-lowering effects, the tablets must be taken at the beginning of meals. In general, the resulting overall glycemic reduction is modest, with A1C changes of 0.5–1.0%. Acarbose is largely not absorbed from the intestine, while miglitol is. The major adverse effects are flatulence, abdominal distress or distension, and diarrhea. These result from excessive blockade of carbohydrate absorption in the small bowel, leading to fermentation and gas production in the colon. They are minimized by a low initial dosage with gradual titration upward. Intestinal distension or diarrhea may be harmful in the presence of inflammatory bowel disease or other major intestinal disorders. There are tantalizing data to suggest that acarbose through unclear mechanisms may be associated with a modest reduction in cardiovascular events.

With the α-glucosidase inhibitors, a program analogous to that described with metformin should be initiated starting with the smallest available tablet once daily with the first bite of the largest meal. Every 2–4 weeks, an additional tablet can be added until the drug is taken at each main meal. Subsequently, the dose of the tablet can be increased, but analogously to the sulfonylureas, there is rarely a substantial response with regard to efficacy as the highest doses are approached, whereas the adverse effects generally worsen proportionately with the dose. Generally, 50 mg three times daily will provide a maximal effect.

Agents Augmenting the Supply of Insulin

Sulfonylureas and non-sulfonylurea insulin secretagogues. Sulfonylureas and non-sulfonylurea insulin secretagogues exert their antidiabetic effects through their interaction with a cell surface protein on the β-cell in pancreatic islets of Langerhans. This protein is termed the "sulfonylurea receptor" (SUR) and regulates the activity of an ATP-dependent potassium channel. Binding of sulfonylureas and non-sulfonylurea secretagogues results in closure of the potassium channel and depolarization of the membrane, with subsequent opening of a calcium channel and stimulation of insulin release. In the β-cell, binding of insulin secretagogues increases insulin secretion in a relatively glucose-independent fashion, resulting in a reduction of fasting glucose as well as a proportional reduction of the postprandial rise of glucose. The net effect is generally a 1–2% reduction in A1C, with the exception being nateglinide, which is associated with a 0.5 to 1% reduction as a result of its short half-life and residence time on the SUR.

The main complication of sulfonylurea treatment is hypoglycemia. Elderly patients are more susceptible, especially when they have declining renal function or tend to skip meals. The risk of hypoglycemia seems to be related to both the pharmacologic half-life as well as the details of the interaction of the drug with the SUR. Glyburide seems to be associated with a higher risk of hypoglycemia than glimepiride, repaglinide, nateglinide, and sustained release formulations of glipizide. In patients with modest hyperglycemia, starting with the lowest possible dose is an important safety consideration to avoid hypoglycemia.

Other side effects are uncommon, but include gastrointestinal symptoms, such as nausea and vomiting, and skin reactions, including rashes, purpura, and pruritis. Rare side effects include hematological reactions (leukopenia, thrombocytopenia, or hemolytic anemia) and cholestasis (with or without jaundice). Modest weight gain may occur when treatment is started.

Some features of the sulfonylureas now available in the United States are shown in Table 3.9. The first-generation sulfonylureas (tolbutamide, tolazamide, and chlorpropamide) bind significantly to plasma proteins and have high milligram dosage requirements. Because of the protein binding, they can displace or be displaced by other agents, such as salicylates or warfarin, leading to drug interactions. Tolbutamide is rapidly cleared by the liver and must be taken two to three times daily. Chlorpropamide is slowly cleared by the kidney and accumulates, particularly when renal function declines, and as a result may cause serious hypoglycemia. Chlorpropamide also may cause an antabuse (disulfiram)-like intolerance to alcohol, or potentiate antidiuretic hormone action leading to water intoxication. Because of these limitations, use of these first-generation agents is uncommon.

The second-generation sulfonylureas (glyburide, glipizide, and glimepiride) are largely free of interactions with other drugs and have lower total dosage requirements. They are metabolized mainly by the liver and cleared renally, except that glimepiride is excreted by both renal and hepatic mechanisms. Glyburide has an active metabolite that must be excreted by the kidney. Thus, in the setting of renal insufficiency, glyburide is associated with greater concern and glimepiride with the least issues from a drug metabolism perspective. Both glyburide and glipizide require twice-daily dosage to produce 24-h coverage. Glipizide is available in an extended-release formulation that along with glimepiride is fully effective given once a day.

The newest insulin secretagogues are non-sulfonylurea agents. Their action is mediated through the SUR, and they hold some structural homology to the sulfonylureas but do not contain the actual sulfonylurea moiety. Both repaglinide and nateglinide are rapidly absorbed after oral administration and rapidly cleared by hepatic metabolism. This rapid time course of action calls for two or three doses daily with meals. Repaglinide is able to reduce fasting levels of glucose despite its short half-life because of prolonged residence on the SUR complex and thus is able to reduce A1C equivalently to sulfonylureas. Nateglinide on the other hand has a short residence time and does not substantially reduce fasting glucose. As a result, nateglinide is the secretagogue with the most specific activity to lower postprandial glucose and lowest risk of hypoglycemia. However, because of its lack of effect on fasting glucose, its efficacy in lowering A1C is modest.

Whether insulin secretagogues that work through the SUR have significant effects beyond the β-cell has been debated. After chronic sulfonylurea treatment, the peripheral tissues can become more sensitive to insulin, but this seems largely due to waning of the adverse effects of hyperglycemia (glucotoxicity). Sulfonylureas bind to potassium channels in various tissues, including vascular tissue, and may reduce vasodilation. Whether this effect is clinically important is unknown. There have been studies suggesting the possibility that sulfonylureas could adversely affect cardiac rhythm in the setting of ischemia. This seems to be less of a concern

Table 3.9 Characteristics of Sulfonylureas

Generic Name	Brand Name	Approved Daily Dosage Range (mg)	Near Maximum Effective Dosage (mg)	Duration of Action (h)	Clearance
Tolbutamide	Orinase	500–3,000	1,000 t.i.d.	6–12	Hepatic
Chlorpropamide	Diabinese	100–500	500 once	>48	Renal
Tolazamide	Tolinase	100–1,000	500 b.i.d.	12–24	Hepatic, renal
Glipizide	Glucotrol	2.5–40	10 b.i.d.	12–18	Hepatic
	Glucotrol XL (extended release)	2.5–20	10 once	24	Hepatic
Glyburide	DiaBeta	1.25–20	5 b.i.d.	12–24	Hepatic
	Micronase	1.25–2	5 b.i.d.	12–24	Hepatic, renal
	Glynase	0.75–12	3 b.i.d.	12–24	Hepatic, renal
Glimepiride	Amaryl	1–8	4 once	24	Hepatic or renal
Repaglinide	Prandin	1–16	4 t.i.d.	2–6	Hepatic
Nateglinide	Starlix	60–360	120 t.i.d	2–4	Hepatic, renal

with glimepiride, with sustained release preparations of glipizide, and with the non-sulfonylurea secretagogues repaglinide and nateglinide than with glyburide. The UKPDS showed no increase in CVD events with sulfonylureas compared with other therapies.

INSULINS

Although insulin has been used therapeutically for over 70 years, some aspects of its use are new. Insulins extracted from the pancreases of cattle and pigs are no longer generally available. They have largely been replaced by insulin that is synthesized by genetically altered bacteria or yeast and that is structurally identical to human insulin as well as insulin analogs in which amino acid substitutions and additions produce altered pharmacokinetics upon subcutaneous injection (Table 3.10). In addition to regular human insulin, NPH human insulin is still available. There are now five structurally modified variants of human insulin, so-called insulin analogs, approved by the U.S. Food and Drug Administration. Three are rapid-acting insulin analogs. Insulin lispro, aspart, and glulisine each involve modifications that disrupt the "tail structure" of the insulin molecule. As a result, these forms of insulin do not exhibit as great a tendency to form dimers and hexamers at high concentrations. The net effect is that these analogs are more rapidly absorbed

Table 3.10 Characteristics of Human Insulins and Analogs in Type 2 Diabetes

		Timing of Action		
Preparation	Trade Name	Onset	Peak	Duration
Rapid-acting				
Lispro, aspart, glulisine	Humalog, Novolog Apidra	<15 minutes	0.5–1.5 h	3–6 h
Short-acting				
Regular	Humulin R Novolin R	30–60 minutes	2–3 h	5–12 h
Intermediate-acting				
NPH	Humulin N Novolin N	2–4 h	6–10 h	10–16 h
Long-acting				
Glargine	Lantus	~2 h	No consistent peak	20–24 h
Detemir	Levemir	~2 h	No consistent peak	12–24 h
Mixtures				
70/30, 50/50, 75/25	Various	30 minutes	7–12 h	16–18 h

Summary of the typical time course of various insulin preparations. These values are highly variable among individuals. Even in a given person, these values vary depending on the site and depth of injection, skin temperature, and exercise, among other factors. Adapted from American Diabetes Association: *Practical Insulin: A Handbook for Providers.* 2nd ed. Alexandria, VA, American Diabetes Association, 2007.

after subcutaneous injection compared with regular insulin, starting to work in 5–15 minutes, peaking in 30–60 minutes, with an effective duration of action of 36 h. Whereas regular human insulin should ideally be administered 30–45 minutes before meals, these analogs should be administered just before meals, or can be given after meals when the size of the meal is not known before eating. These rapid-acting insulin analogs are associated with a somewhat lower risk of hypoglycemia with similar or slightly greater improvements in A1C compared with regular insulin.

There are two long-acting insulin analogs. Glargine insulin has been modified to form a precipitate at neutral pH. It is supplied as a clear colorless solution at acidic pH and upon subcutaneous injection precipitates with slow dissolution, producing essentially peakless action over ~24 h. Studies have demonstrated that in patients failing oral agents, administration of glargine once nightly compared with NPH insulin is associated with identical overall glycemic control, as assessed by A1C, but with a lower risk of hypoglycemia, particularly during the night. Insulin detemir has a fatty acid side chain that binds to albumin, providing for prolonged duration of action. There is some evidence that weight gain associated with initiation of insulin therapy may be less with detemir insulin. The basis for the effect is unknown.

Premixed combinations of insulins are now available and in wide use. The forms available in the United States are 70/30 (70% NPH and 30% regular) and 50/50 (50% NPH and 50% regular) human insulin as well as mixtures of analogs.

Insulin has essentially unlimited power to reduce plasma glucose. It reduces the blood glucose level by suppressing hepatic glucose production and by increasing glucose uptake by insulin-sensitive tissues, notably muscle and adipose tissue. As with sulfonylureas, the improved glycemic control achieved with insulin therapy generally increases the responsiveness of tissues to insulin. The main practical limitation in achieving treatment objectives with insulin is the risk of hypoglycemia. Also, patients with type 2 diabetes, who are typically already obese, usually gain weight when insulin treatment is started. Other side effects include immediate skin reactions at injection sites (itching, redness, and swelling) or persistent lumps or swelling at these sites that may represent delayed hypersensitivity reactions. These allergy-related problems are less common with current insulin preparations than with previous ones and may be less common in people with type 2 diabetes than in people with type 1 diabetes.

Agents Modifying Non-Insulin Hormonal Systems

Amylinomimetics. Amylin is a neuroendocrine hormone co-secreted with insulin by pancreatic β-cells. As would be expected, amylin deficiency is evident in type 1 diabetes. In type 2 diabetes, amylin levels may be fairly high in the fasting state but do not increase with meals as robustly as in non-diabetes. Amylin and insulin have complementary actions in regulating plasma glucose. Amylin binds to brain nuclei and through central mechanisms promotes satiety, reduces appetite, decreases the rate of gastric emptying, and suppresses glucagon secretion in a glucose-dependent fashion. The net effect of amylin secretion is to regulate the rate of glucose appearance from the gastrointestinal tract and the liver. Insulin on the other hand regulates the rate of glucose disappearance from the circulation by stimulating glucose uptake in muscle and fat.

However, amylin is relatively insoluble in aqueous solution and aggregates on plastic and glass. Pramlintide was developed as a soluble, nonaggregating, equipotent amylin analog. It is indicated for use in type 1 diabetes and insulin-treated patients with type 2 diabetes for mealtime subcutaneous injection. In type 2 diabetic patients treated with insulin either alone or in combination with metformin and/or sulfonylurea, addition of pramlintide, 120-μg injections, before meals reduced A1C by ~0.4% and weight by ~2 kg over 52 weeks compared with placebo. Mild nausea, which wanes with continued therapy, is the most common adverse effect; it is minimized by titrating from 60 μg with meals to the usual 120-μg dose over 3–7 days as tolerated. Hypoglycemia is less frequent in type 2 diabetes than in patients with type 1 diabetes who do occasionally exhibit severe hypoglycemia; nevertheless, the suggestion to reduce prandial insulin by 50% when initiating therapy is recommended in both clinical situations. Oral medications that require rapid absorption for effectiveness should be administered either 1 h before or 2 h after injection of pramlintide.

Incretin-related therapies. The incretins are hormones that mediate the effects of oral glucose (i.e., a greater stimulatory effect on insulin secretion than intravenous glucose when the same level of circulating glucose is achieved). In humans, this effect seems to be primarily driven by GLP-1 and glucose-dependent insulinotropic peptide (GIP). GLP-1 is produced from the proglucagon gene in intestinal L-cells and is secreted in response to nutrients. GLP-1 stimulates insulin secretion and inhibits hyperglucagonemia in the setting of hyperglycemia, slows gastric emptying, reduces appetite, and improves satiety. In animal models of diabetes, GLP-1 has been demonstrated to have proliferative, anti-apoptotic, and differentiation effects on β-cells, but no evidence is available from humans. GLP-1 has a very short half-life in plasma of 1–2 minutes because of N-terminal degradation by the enzyme dipeptidyl peptidase IV (DPP-4). A variety of pharmacologic techniques have been developed to harness the potential of incretins to treat diabetes. These include incretin mimetics, GLP-1 analogs, and DPP-4 inhibition.

Exendin-4 is a naturally occurring component of the saliva of the Gila monster (*Heloderma suspectum*), shares 53% sequence identity with GLP-1, and is resistant to DPP-4 degradation. Exenatide is synthetic exendin-4 and was the first GLP-1–based therapy to be approved for human use in the U.S. When injected subcutaneously, it has a peak of action and half-life of ~2 h. Because of the pharmacokinetics of exenatide in its current formulation, its effects are largely postprandial without marked effect in the fasting state. It is indicated for the treatment of patients with type 2 diabetes inadequately controlled on metformin and/or sulfonylurea therapy. At a dose of 10 μg injected subcutaneously twice daily, A1C is reduced ~1% with ~1/2 to 1 lb per month of weight loss compared with placebo. Open-label extension studies have demonstrated sustained lowering of A1C and progressive weight loss averaging ~12 lb at 2 years. With prolonged use, weight loss has been associated with expected improvements in blood pressure, lipids, C-reactive protein, and liver transaminases.

The most common adverse effect of exenatide is nausea, which occurs in 40–50% of patients, generally early in the course of therapy, mild to moderate in intensity, and waning over time. Gastrointestinal adverse effects lead to withdrawal of therapy in ~5% of patients. Nausea is reduced in intensity by dose titration. The recommendation is that therapy begin with 5 μg injected subcutaneously twice daily for the first month with titration to 10 μg twice daily as tolerated. Initially, dosing immediately before meals reduces nausea; with time, spreading the injection to 30–60 minutes before meals seems to increase weight loss. Although hypoglycemia does not occur at higher rates than seen with placebo when exenatide is combined with metformin and/or glitazones, mild to moderate hypoglycemia can be observed in combination with sulfonylureas. Prospectively reducing the dose of sulfonylureas to the smallest available tablet size reduces hypoglycemia without substantially sacrificing efficacy. Rare cases of pancreatitis have been reported, although it is uncertain that exenatide is etiologic; abdominal pain with sustained nausea and vomiting should be evaluated in a patient on exenatide with this possibility in mind.

Numerous DPP-4 inhibitors are being developed for human use. Sitagliptin is the first DPP-4 inhibitor available for treatment of type 2 diabetes. It produces an approximately twofold increase in GLP-1 and GIP and is associated with A1C reduction of ~0.7%, whether used as monotherapy or in combination with metformin, sulfonylureas, or glitazones. Sitagliptin is not associated with weight loss or nausea.

A DPP-IV–resistant analog of GLP-1, liraglutide, is now in phase 3 trials. With once-daily subcutaneous injection, it is associated with similar efficacy on A1C and weight as exenatide, although with greater lowering of fasting glucose and less nausea. A once-weekly formulation of exenatide is also in phase 3 trials. Many other DPP-IV inhibitors and GLP-1 analogs are under development.

Algorithm of Care

With more agents to choose from, pharmacotherapy of type 2 diabetes has become both more effective and more complex over the last decade (Fig. 3.1). Different agents have unique clinical effects (Table 3.8). The first treatment decision is required when a patient is found, despite the best possible effort with lifestyle modification, to have an A1C level >7% or consistently elevated fasting glucose levels. The UKPDS demonstrated that 10-year average A1C values of ~7% were associated with better outcomes than average A1C values of 8%. The treatment protocol in the UKPDS held that if a patient had a fasting glucose >108 mg/dl, he or she was eligible for randomization. Those patients randomized to continue on lifestyle intervention had poorer outcomes than those randomized to medications. Thus, the evidence would suggest that drug therapy is indicated if fasting glucose cannot be controlled to levels <108 mg/dl, despite best lifestyle efforts for 3 months. There are no similar trials that provide cut points for postprandial glucose levels associated with improved outcomes.

Recently, the American Diabetes Association published a consensus statement titled "Management of Hyperglycemia in Type 2 Diabetes." It suggested that because of the high failure of lifestyle therapy to maintain glucose control over time and because of the excellent performance of metformin in pre-diabetic individuals in the Diabetes Prevention Program (DPP), the initial therapy of patients with diabetes should include both lifestyle intervention plus metformin titrated to the maximal effective dose (1,000 mg twice daily) over 1–2 months. If that is insufficient to control glucose or maintain control adequately, three second-line therapies are recommended:

- Basal insulin (NPH, glargine, or detemir) titrated to control fasting glucose to 70–130 mg/dl). This therapy is highlighted as the most effective approach and is particularly appropriate in patients with symptomatic hyperglycemia, fasting glucose >250 mg/dl, postprandial glucose >300 mg/dl, or A1C >10%.
- Sulfonylureas. This therapy is highlighted as the least expensive option, but can lead to hypoglycemia.
- Thiazolidinediones. This therapy is highlighted for providing glucose lowering without risk of hypoglycemia; an update to the original publication of the ADA/EASD treatment algorithm (Nathan DM, et al. 2006) points out that pioglitazone is associated with improved lipid profile and potential decrease in cardiovascular events, and rosiglitazone is associated with a potential increase in cardiovascular events. The updated statement also discusses the risks of congestive heart failure and fractures with both agents.

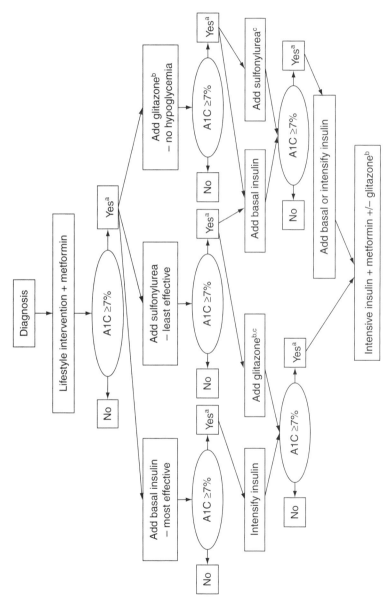

Figure 3.1 Algorithm for the metabolic management of type 2 diabetes. Reinforce lifestyle intervention at every visit. [a]Check A1C every 3 months until <7% and then at least every 6 months. [b]Associated with increased risk of fluid retention, coronary heart failure, and fractures. Rosiglitazone, but probably not pioglitazone, may be associated with an increased risk of myocardial infarction. [c]Although three oral agents can be used, initiation and intensification of insulin therapy is preferred based on effectiveness and lower expense. From Nathan et al., 2008.

Other agents listed in Tables 3.7 and 3.8 are not highlighted in the algorithm because they are in general less well established as safe and effective in long-term outcome studies. Furthermore, as a group, these agents are associated with lesser glycemic efficacy, greater adverse effects, or greater expense. That said, all of these agents have lowered A1C and, in general, are more active in the postprandial period and less likely to produce weight gain. They may be appropriate in individual patients.

FPG <130 mg/dl. Patients with relatively modest elevations of FPG who require A1C reduction arguably should be preferentially treated with agents not associated with hypoglycemic risk. Metformin may be the best studied agent of this type for the treatment of diabetes. As discussed above, it is not associated with weight gain and was associated with reduced mortality among overweight patients randomized in the UKPDS. The glitazone agents are generally better tolerated, although more expensive and less well studied. The α-glucosidase inhibitors are not associated with hypoglycemia or weight gain, but have not been well accepted in our society because of cultural stigma regarding the most common adverse effect—flatulence. That said, there is substantial reason to believe that these agents are advantageous and should be considered. Nateglinide among the secretagogues has the lowest potential for severe hypoglycemia and would be a reasonable choice, particularly in patients with near-normal fasting glucose. Exenatide and sitagliptin likewise are not associated with hypoglycemia. Extended-release glipizide or glimepiride or another sulfonylurea could be tried at the lowest possible dose, although many patients will have symptomatic hypoglycemia at least intermittently. Finally, insulin therapy is not out of the question at this level of glycemic control, although it would rarely be the leading choice of many patients or providers.

FPG >130 mg/dl. When FPG is >130 mg/dl, the aforementioned options will also apply. Although in general, the ability of the more postprandially targeted oral approaches (α-glucosidase inhibitors, nateglinide, exenatide, and pramlintide) will often not produce adequate overall control in large measure because they do not exert enough glucose-lowering action through the night.

Sulfonylureas are much less likely to be associated with substantial problems with frequent or severe hypoglycemia in this scenario, particularly if starting with a low dose. The dose of a sulfonylurea can be increased with just a few days of experience, since they work very quickly at maximal effect. Maximal clinical effectiveness is usually reached at half the maximal labeled dose of sulfonylureas.

Consideration can also be given to initiating two agents in this setting, particularly if the A1C is >9% or fasting glucose is >200 mg/dl, since a single agent will not usually produce an adequate reduction in glucose. In general, the combination of agents that improve insulin action (metformin, glitazones, or α-glucosidase inhibitors) with agents that increase insulin levels (secretagogues, exenatide, sitagliptin, insulin) will be more potent in reducing A1C than other combinations.

However, the combinations of metformin with a glitazone or metformin with sitagliptin are quite compelling, in that there should be very low risk of hypoglycemia or weight gain. There are several tablets that combine oral antidiabetic agents (metformin plus glitazone, metformin plus sitagliptin, metformin plus sulfonylurea, glitazone plus sulfonylurea). They provide substantial convenience and perhaps the potential for better adherence, but do provide somewhat less flexibility in dosing and dose adjustment.

Insulin may also be used for initial treatment or at any point during the course of type 2 diabetes, although most patients prefer to use oral treatments first. In symptomatic patients or those with very poor glycemic control, there should be no hesitation to start insulin therapy. Oral agents can be added later and an effort made to withdraw insulin if that is the patient's and provider's desire. It is important to remember that in patients presenting with weight loss or ketonuria or who have a poor response to initial therapy with oral agents, it is possible if not likely that they have type 1 rather than type 2 diabetes.

Management with insulin during pregnancy or surgery is discussed under the topic "Special Therapeutic Situations."

When insulin is started by patients not taking oral agents, a single injection of intermediate-acting or long-acting insulin may be given either before breakfast or at bedtime. Patients with predominantly daytime hyperglycemia who start the day with a reasonable fasting glucose that rises with each meal may respond better to a morning injection. The more common pattern is dominated by fasting hyperglycemia, and these patients are better candidates for a bedtime injection. In randomized trials, the evening insulin approach in the setting of type 2 diabetes has generally been associated with better control and less weight gain.

For the average overweight uncontrolled patient, a conservative starting dose of 10 units at bedtime is unlikely to cause hypoglycemia, yet will improve glycemia somewhat while the patient is learning to handle and inject insulin. Glucose monitoring by SMBG should be done at least every morning, with occasional monitoring at other times of the day to determine if glucose levels rise during the day and if there is unrecognized hypoglycemia. A recent study demonstrated that a simple algorithm to drive once-weekly titration of bedtime NPH or glargine works well with professional supervision. In the Treat to Target study, if there was no fasting glucose <72 mg/dl, no severe hypoglycemia, and no glucose <56 mg/dl documented in the prior week, the average of the prior 2 days' fasting glucose was used to drive the increase. If it was >180 mg/dl, the bedtime dose was increased by 8 units/day. If the average was 140–180 mg/dl, the dose was increased by 6 units. If the average was 120–140 mg/dl, the dose was increased by 4 units, and if between 100 and 120 mg/dl, the dose was increased 2 units. An alternative approach is to ask patients to increase their dose of insulin by 1 unit daily whenever the fasting glucose is >100 mg/dl and decrease it by 2–4 units for glucose levels <70 mg/dl, until most fasting glucose levels are in the target range of 70–130 mg/dl.

Table 3.11 provides some additional considerations for monitoring if bedtime insulin is not the initial regimen prescribed.

Some patients will have excellent responses with a single insulin injection and may maintain target levels of control this way for some time. In other cases, two or more daily injections will be required for best results. If a patient started with long- or intermediate-acting insulin at bedtime, often a second injection of rapid-acting or regular insulin is given with the largest meal of the day or the meal with the greatest glycemic excursion, which is usually breakfast or dinner. The formerly traditional so-called split-mixed insulin at breakfast and dinner has become less popular recently since the advent of premixed insulin formulations and the availability of insulin pens. Some prefer to start with such a regimen without a trial of long- or intermediate-acting insulin at bedtime. In this scenario, generally, a mixture of intermediate- and rapid-acting or regular insulins should be given before

Table 3.11 Insulin Regimen and Timing of Self-Monitoring of Blood Glucose

Insulin	Time Injected	Period of Greatest Activity	SMBG Reflecting Insulin Action
Rapid-acting	Just before or after the meal	After the meal	1–2 h after injection or just before the next meal
Regular	Before a meal	Between that meal and the next meal or bedtime	Just before the next meal; occasionally 1–2 h after injection
Intermediate-acting	Before breakfast	Between lunch and evening meal	Before lunch and dinner
	Before evening meal	Between midnight and breakfast	Before bedtime, midsleep, and breakfast
	At bedtime	Between 4:00 a.m. and breakfast	Before breakfast
Long-acting	Before breakfast or bedtime	Mostly overnight, because short-acting insulin overrides its effect during the day	Before breakfast

The table shows the times at which different kinds of injected insulin are most active in reducing glucose levels when given at various times of day. Rapid-acting insulin is given before meals and is active up to 3 h, but with large injections up to 6 h after the meal. Regular insulin is generally active for 6 h and can be active for 12 or more hours with large injections. Intermediate-acting insulin has peak activity 6–12 h after injection. Because intermediate-acting insulin is commonly given before breakfast, before the evening meal, or at bedtime, it may cause hypoglycemia in the late afternoon, from midnight to 4:00 a.m., or just before breakfast.

breakfast and before the evening meal (Fig. 3.2). The ratio of the morning to evening doses needed varies among patients. Some need up to two-thirds of the total in the morning, others need two-thirds in the evening, and many need approximately equal amounts at each injection. The same is true of the ratio of intermediate- to rapid-acting or regular insulin at each dose. Some patients do very well with a 2-to-1 ratio; others do better with a 1-to-1 ratio. A simple and reasonable way to begin two-injection treatment is with 10 units of premixed or self-mixed insulin twice daily. Both the dosage and distribution should be modified as indicated by the SMBG results. Relatively nonobese patients may achieve good glucose control with no more than 20–40 units daily. More obese patients will need more, often 100–200 units daily. Occasionally, patients will need to mix intermediate- and short-acting insulins from separate vials to vary the ratio for optimal results.

A multiple daily injection (MDI) regimen, analogous to the techniques commonly used in type 1 diabetes, provides the greatest flexibility on the part of the patient. With the advent of insulin pens, MDI is convenient, even with the most active lifestyles (Fig. 3.3). MDI is generally required in two circumstances: for hypoglycemia with activity or delayed meals, or for rising glucose levels during the

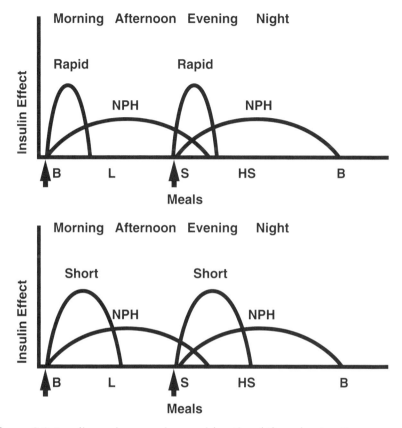

Figure 3.2 Insulin regimens using rapid-acting (*A*) or short-acting (*B*) insulin with NPH insulin. From *Practical Insulin: A Handbook for Providers.* 2nd ed. Alexandria, VA, American Diabetes Association, 2007.

day, despite achieving adequate control of fasting glucose. In transitioning from one injection to two or more, there is one very important safety consideration. If the patient's fasting glucose is well controlled, great care should be taken as the second or subsequent injection is added to avoid the development of nocturnal or morning hypoglycemia. In such circumstances, it is prudent to reduce the long-acting insulin dose by 10–25% or an amount at least as great as the rapid-acting insulin added.

Second, patients should be reminded of the relationship between carbohydrate intake and meal-related insulin requirements. The insulin regimen that provides for excellent glycemic control after a breakfast of cereal and juice will certainly result in hypoglycemia after bacon and eggs. Two techniques for dealing with this relationship include setting a fixed intake of carbohydrate at each main meal or using the technique of carbohydrate counting. In the latter, patients are instructed to count either servings or grams of carbohydrates in their meals and are provided

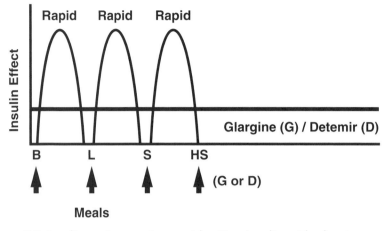

Figure 3.3 Insulin regimen using rapid-acting insulin with glargine or detemir. From *Practical Insulin: A Handbook for Providers.* 2nd ed. Alexandria, VA, American Diabetes Association, 2007.

with a ratio of insulin to administer per serving or gram of carbohydrates. Generally, starting at 1 unit per carbohydrate serving or 1 unit per 15 g carbohydrates is reasonable. Most patients with type 2 diabetes will require 2–5 units per 15-g serving of carbohydrates. There are many available carbohydrate-counting guides to assist in this process. Patients generally rapidly adapt to this technique because the number of food choices that most patients will consume over a period of weeks is remarkably limited, and they quickly master the carbohydrate content of foods consumed.

In patients with type 2 diabetes, injections with each meal may not be needed. As an example, a patient may do well on a regimen of long-acting insulin at bedtime with a rapid-acting insulin analog at breakfast in the setting of a carbohydrate-rich breakfast but be able to avoid an injection at lunch if it is modest in carbohydrate content and the patient is active during the day. Some patients will only require rapid-acting insulin with dinner. The advantages of this technique are numerous, since it provides great flexibility and also highlights the relationship of dietary intake with glycemic control.

It is worth mentioning that continuous insulin infusion or insulin pump therapy is an alternative to insulin injection in the setting of type 2 diabetes. Studies to date have not demonstrated the superiority of insulin pump therapy, particularly in type 2 diabetes. However, for some patients whose dietary habit is to graze during the day and who have difficulty adhering to administering insulin with each snack, it is remarkable how much more effective pump therapy can be, because it allows patients to quickly and conveniently administer insulin an unlimited number of times during the day as they eat.

Insulin after failure of oral agents. The task of starting insulin is slightly different when oral agents have been used previously and secondary failure has ensued. There are two options. The first and traditional option is to stop oral agents and begin insulin alone. However, after secondary failure of oral agents, insulin must be used more aggressively than when it is the initial treatment. The reason for this is that by the time secondary failure of oral agents has occurred, the underlying defects of insulin secretion and action have progressed, and withdrawing oral agents may lead to rapid loss of glycemic control.

Previously, many believed that a single injection of insulin was unlikely to be effective, and two injections should be started immediately, at a dosage of 10–15 units twice daily. On the other hand, the Treat to Target study above did demonstrate that >50% of the time, patients failing one or two oral agents were able to achieve an A1C of <7% with one injection of bedtime NPH or glargine. It should be noted that these patients' glucose levels throughout the course of the day were not normal, although, in many patients, average glucose levels over months were sufficiently low to reach the A1C goal. The dosage should be increased at frequent intervals, guided by the results of SMBG.

In general, it is simpler and arguably more effective to add insulin to the prior oral regimen. Again, available clinical trial data suggest that once-daily glargine, NPH at bedtime, or, in more obese patients, premixed insulin before the evening meal is more effective than alternative approaches. The rationale is that supplementing with overnight insulin will control fasting hyperglycemia, whereas continuing the oral agents will prevent worsening of glycemic control during the time that the insulin dosage is titrated upward.

LONG-TERM COMBINATIONS OF ORAL AGENTS WITH INSULIN

By the time oral agents have failed, β-cell function has usually declined enough that sulfonylureas provide little benefit and can be stopped. It should be noted that occasional patients are able to maintain glycemic control better through the day when on regimens involving morning sulfonylureas versus having just a single injection of insulin at night. Studies have demonstrated that the degree of glucose lowering is on average greater when insulin is added to a glitazone than when insulin is used alone. Insulin plus metformin is associated with lesser weight gain than when insulin is used alone. Certainly, the continued use of oral agents can reduce the total insulin dosage, sometimes preventing the need to use more than a single 100-unit syringe-full at a given time of day. For these reasons, continuing the agents enhancing insulin action may be given serious consideration.

The effect of combining metformin, glitazones, or sulfonylureas with insulin is best seen when one of these agents is either added to or withdrawn from a previously established insulin treatment. There are occasional patients who are treated with insulin alone, having never received metformin or a glitazone. In such patients, perhaps one-third to one-half can be withdrawn from insulin on combined oral agent therapy by reducing the dose of insulin sequentially by 10–25% while oral agents are titrated in and glucose levels remain in the target range.

ADJUSTING INSULIN DOSAGE
IN LONG-TERM TYPE 2 DIABETES

By 10 years after the onset of type 2 diabetes, most patients will have markedly reduced endogenous insulin secretion. At this time, glycemic variability increases and reliance on injected insulin becomes greater. Therefore, treatment of these patients becomes more like that of type 1 diabetes than it was earlier in the course of their type 2 diabetes. Both the patient and the physician must be aware of the time course of action of the various kinds of insulin and the times at which hypoglycemia is most likely to occur. Blood glucose levels must be monitored at home regularly by the patient or a responsible helper, and adjustments of meal pattern and/or insulin should be made when necessary.

Different insulin regimens are shown in Table 3.12. The once- and twice-daily regimens were discussed in some detail above. Both are quite effective for the vast majority of patients with type 2 diabetes. The dosages used at each injection can be adjusted on the basis of SMBG results. Disproportionately high values before lunch suggest inadequate rapid-acting or regular insulin in the morning injection, and high values at bedtime suggest the rapid-acting or regular insulin before the evening meal is insufficient. Similarly, high glucose readings before the evening meal or breakfast suggest that the need to increase the morning or evening intermediate-acting dose in the two-injection regimens and the long-acting insulin in the one-injection regimen (unless an injection is provided at lunch). Low glucose values suggest excessive dosage of the insulins responsible for coverage at each of these times of day. When adjustments of individual components of the insulin regimen are necessary, premixed insulins (70/30 or 50/50) are less effective, and better results will be obtained if the patient mixes the insulins for each injection.

Some patients who take intermediate-acting insulin at dinner will be bothered by nocturnal hypoglycemia and/or inadequate control of the fasting glucose. A switch to analog long-acting insulin (glargine or detemir) insulin or moving the

Table 3.12 Sample Insulin Regimens for Achieving Glycemic Control

Injections	Before Breakfast	Before Lunch	Before Dinner	Bedtime
1				Intermediate- or long-acting
	Regular or rapid-acting			Intermediate- or long-acting
			Regular or rapid-acting	Intermediate- or long-acting
2		Regular or rapid-acting		Intermediate- or long-acting
	Intermediate-acting + Regular or rapid-acting		Intermediate-acting + Regular or rapid-acting	
	Regular or rapid-acting		Regular or rapid-acting	Intermediate- or long-acting
3	Intermediate-acting + Regular or rapid-acting		Regular or rapid-acting	Intermediate-acting
4	Regular or rapid-acting	Regular or rapid-acting	Regular or rapid-acting	Intermediate- or long-acting

intermediate-acting insulin to bedtime will generally remedy that situation. In general, long-acting analogs have been demonstrated to have moderately lower rates of nocturnal hypoglycemia and in some instances less weight gain than NPH insulin. The advantage of moving the intermediate-acting insulin to bedtime is to reduce the chance of hypoglycemia between midnight and 4:00 a.m. by shifting the peak effect of intermediate-acting insulin closer to breakfast. This change is necessary mostly for active, less obese patients who absorb insulin rapidly and may develop nocturnal hypoglycemia on the two-injection regimen.

Three- and four-shot regimens are technically MDI regimens that may be desirable for patients who tend to have more variable SMBG readings. Generally, the more injections that are provided, the greater the flexibility the patient will have regarding the content and timing of meals and activity as well as the lower the glycemic excursions. Individualized regimens may be required as determined by meal patterns or by SMBG results. For example, some older people awaken late and eat just two meals—the first (and sometimes main) meal close to midday and a second meal in the evening. In this case, the first insulin injection may best be given before the midday meal and the second before the evening meal.

BIBLIOGRAPHY

Amori RE, Lau J, Pittas AG: Efficacy and safety of incretin therapy in type 2 diabetes: systematic review and meta-analysis. *JAMA* 298:194–206, 2007

Bolen S, Feldman L, Vassy J, Wilson L, Yeh HC, Marinopoulos S, Wiley C, Selvin E, Wilson R, Bass EB, Brancati FL: Systematic review: comparative effectiveness and safety of oral medications for type 2 diabetes mellitus. *Ann Intern Med* 147:386–390, 2007

Buse JB, Polonsky KS, Burant CF: Type 2 diabetes mellitus. In *Williams Textbook of Endocrinology.* 11th ed. Kronenberg HM, Melmed S, Polonsky KS, Larsen PR, Eds. Philadelphia, PA, Elsevier Science, 2008, p. 1329–1389

Chiquette E, Ramirez G, DeFronzo R: A meta-analysis comparing the effect of thiazolidinediones on cardiovascular risk factors. *Arch Intern Med* 164:2097–2104, 2004

Dormandy JA, Charbonnel B, Eckland DJ, Erdmann E, Massi-Benedetti M, Moules IK, Skene AM, Tan MH, Lefebvre PJ, Murray GD, Standl E, Wilcox RG, Wilhelmsen L, Betteridge J, Birkeland K, Golay A, Heine RJ, Koranyi L, Laakso M, Mokan M, Norkus A, Pirags V, Podar T, Scheen A, Scherbaum W, Schernthaner G, Schmitz O, Skrha J, Smith U, Taton J, PROactive Investigators: Secondary prevention of macrovascular events in patients with type 2 diabetes in the PROactive Study (PROspective pioglitAzone Clinical Trial In macrovascular Events): a randomised controlled trial. *Lancet* 366:1279–1289, 2005

Dornhorst A: Insulinotropic meglitinide analogues. *Lancet* 358:1709–1716, 2001

Hanefeld M, Cagatay M, Petrowitsch T, Neuser D, Petzinna D, Rupp M: Acarbose reduces the risk for myocardial infarction in type 2 diabetic patients: meta-analysis of seven long-term studies. *Eur Heart J* 25:10–16, 2004

Heine RJ, Van Gaal LF, Johns D, Mihm MJ, Widel MH, Brodows RG, GWAA Study Group: Exenatide versus insulin glargine in patients with suboptimally controlled type 2 diabetes: a randomized trial. *Ann Intern Med* 143:559–569, 2005

Hirsch IB, Richard M, Bergenstal CG, Parkin EW Jr, Buse JB: A real-world approach to insulin therapy in primary care practice. *Clinical Diabetes* 23:78–86, 2005

Holleman F, Gale EA: Nice insulins, pity about the evidence. *Diabetologia* 50:1783–1790, 2007

Karl D, Philis-Tsimikas A, Darsow T, Lorenzi G, Kellmeyer T, Lutz K, Wang Y, Frias JP: Pramlintide as an adjunct to insulin in patients with type 2 diabetes in a clinical practice setting reduced A1C, postprandial glucose excursions, and weight. *Diabetes Technol Ther* 9:191–199, 2007

Kirpichnikov D, McFarlane SI, Sowers JR: Metformin: an update. *Ann Intern Med* 137:25–33, 2002

Lebovitz HE: Alpha-glucosidase inhibitors. *Endocrinol Metab Clin North Am* 26:539–551, 1997

Nathan DM, Buse JB, Davidson MB, Heine RJ, Holman RR, Sherwin R, Zinman B: Management of hyperglycemia in type 2 diabetes: a consensus algorithm for the initiation and adjustment of therapy: a consensus statement from the American Diabetes Association and the European Association for the Study of Diabetes. *Diabetes Care* 29:1963–1972, 2006

Nathan DM, Buse JB, Davidson MB, Ferrannini E, Holman RR, Sherwin R, Zinman B: Management of hyperglycemia in type 2 diabetes: a consensus algorithm for the initiation and adjustment of therapy: update regarding thiazolidinediones: a consensus statement from the American Diabetes Association and the European Association for the Study of Diabetes. *Diabetes Care* 31:173–175, 2008

Nesto RW, Bell D, Bonow RO, Fonseca V, Grudny SM, Horton ES, Le Winter M, Porte D, Semenkovich CF, Smith S, Young LH, Kanh R: Thiazolidinedione use, fluid retention, and congestive heart failure: a consensus statement from the American Heart Association and American Diabetes Association. *Diabetes Care* 27:256–263, 2004

Polonsky WH, Jackson RA: What's so tough about taking insulin? Addressing the problem of psychological insulin resistance in type 2 diabetes. *Clinical Diabetes* 22:147–150, 2004

Raskin P, Bode BW, Marks JB, Hirsch IB, Weinstein RL, McGill JB, Peterson GE, Mudaliar SR, Reinhardt RR: Continuous subcutaneous insulin infusion and multiple daily injection therapy are equally effective in type 2 diabetes: a randomized, parallel-group, 24-week study. *Diabetes Care* 26:2598–2603, 2003

Riddle MC, Rosenstock J, Gerich J, Insulin Glargine 4002 Study Investigators: The Treat-to-Target Trial: randomized addition of glargine or human NPH insulin to oral therapy of type 2 diabetic patients. *Diabetes Care* 26:3080–3086, 2003

Shaw JS, Wilmot RL, Kilpatrick ES: Establishing pragmatic estimated GFR thresholds to guide metformin prescribing. *Diabet Med* 24:1160–1163, 2007

Turner RC, Cull CA, Frighi V, Holman RR: Glycemic control with diet, sulfonylurea, metformin, or insulin in patients with type 2 diabetes mellitus: progressive requirement for multiple therapies (UKPDS 49). *JAMA* 281:2005–2012, 1999

U.K. Prospective Diabetes Study Group: Intensive blood-glucose control with sulphonylureas or insulin compared with conventional treatment and risk of complications in patients with type 2 diabetes (UKPDS 33). *Lancet* 352:837–853, 1998

U.K. Prospective Diabetes Study Group: Effect of intensive blood-glucose control with metformin on complications in overweight patients with type 2 diabetes (UKPDS 34). *Lancet* 352:854–865, 1998

Zimmerman BR: Sulfonylureas. *Endocrinol Metab Clin North Am* 26:511–522, 1997

ASSESSMENT OF TREATMENT EFFICACY

In clinical practice, response to the treatment of type 2 diabetes should be monitored through a schedule of patient interviews and examinations with a comprehensive assessment of:

- Continued patient acceptance of the treatment plan and goals
- Symptoms
- Weight
- Blood pressure
- Smoking
- Screening evaluations for complications, including:
  - Lipid levels
  - Urine microalbumin-to-creatinine ratio
  - Dilated eye exams
  - Comprehensive foot exams
- Various parameters of glycemic control

Among these parameters, glycemic control is unique in that techniques have been developed to allow both the patient and the health care team to independently and synergistically assess the response of glucose metabolism to therapy. This section will focus on assessment of treatment efficacy as reflected in glycemic targets (Table 3.13). In general, providers assess blood glucose control with assays for glycated hemoglobin. Intermittent measurements of fasting, preprandial, and postprandial plasma glucose levels in the office may be useful.

For most patients, SMBG is critical in that it creates a situation in which the patients can be in control of their own therapy. If patients are aware of the glycemic targets associated with the outcomes they seek to achieve, SMBG provides a way for them to critically evaluate their response to therapy and to assure themselves that they are reaching their goals. In this process, it is essential that patients and practitioners agree on mutually acceptable glycemic targets, the frequency and pattern of SMBG, and a plan for interpreting and acting on the results obtained. To this end, it is generally useful for patients to keep a daily diary of their SMBG results, not only so that they can periodically assess their results, but also so they can share them with the health care team. Sometimes recording food intake, activity, symptoms, and doses of diabetes medications simultaneously provides the patient and health care team with a better understanding of the factors that influence the level of glycemic control.

The frequency and type of monitoring of diabetes therapy should be determined in consultation with patients, taking into account the nature of their diabetes, their overall treatment plans and goals, and their abilities. The practitioner should also be aware of the financial burden of SMBG supplies. In many instances, the financial burden can be the limiting factor for compliance with recommended blood glucose monitoring. Recent changes in federal and state insurance regulations are making SMBG a covered benefit for most insured patients. A list of products available for SMBG and their features can be found in the American Diabetes Association's Buyer's Guide to Diabetes Products, an annual supplement found in the January issue of *Diabetes Forecast*. SMBG does require a modicum of manual dexterity, cooperation, and intelligence. With currently available equipment and

Table 3.13 Glycemic Control for People with Diabetes*

A1C	<7.0%*
Preprandial plasma glucose	70–130 mg/dl (3.9–7.2 mmol/l)
Postprandial plasma glucose†	<180 mg/dl (<10.0 mmol/l)

Key concepts in setting glycemic goals:
- A1C is the primary target for glycemic control.
- Goals should be individualized based on duration of diabetes, pregnancy status, age, comorbid conditions, hypoglycemia unawareness, and individual patient considerations.
- More stringent glycemic goals (i.e., a normal A1C, <6%) may further reduce complications at the cost of increased risk of hypoglycemia.
- Postprandial glucose may be targeted if A1C goals are not met despite reaching a preprandial glucose goal.

*Referenced to a nondiabetic range of 4.0–6.0% using a DCCT-based assay. †Postprandial glucose measurements should be made 1–2 h after the beginning of the meal, generally peak levels in patients with diabetes.

established patient education techniques, there are few people who cannot successfully monitor blood glucose at home.

Each of the assessment methods described below has advantages and disadvantages. Most often, a combination of methods is used to determine the degree of metabolic control.

OFFICE METHODS

When patients visit their health care providers, the clinician can assess the degree of blood glucose control with a laboratory venous plasma glucose determination, a capillary plasma glucose determination, and/or an assay for glycated hemoglobin. These measurements are of value in different ways. The venous glucose or capillary glucose is an index of moment-to-moment control and can also be used to compare with simultaneously obtained patient SMBG results to check patient technique as well as the meter's accuracy. Glycated hemoglobin concentration reflects the level of glucose control for the preceding 2–3 months and has been well established through the DCCT, the UKPDS, and other prospective studies, to predict the risk of developing complications. Other glycated serum proteins can be measured in the laboratory but are not as well validated to reflect risk of complications. Each reflects the level of glycemic control over shorter periods of time proportional to their circulating half-life. A relatively new marker, 1,5-anhydroglucitol (1,5-AG), reflects glycemic excursions, often in the postprandial state, more robustly than A1C and may be useful as a complementary marker to A1C to assess glycemic control in moderately controlled patients with diabetes (A1C <8%).

Office Glucose Determinations

Fasting as well as 1- to 2-h postprandial glucose levels are easily measured and useful parameters for determining metabolic control. The major drawback to random plasma glucose determinations, particularly in a patient with moderate to severe disease, is that it is difficult to know what a single blood glucose determination reflects other than the level of glucose at that moment. Blood glucose levels can range widely during the day, so random determinations may represent peak values, trough values, or values in between. Furthermore, if the patient is visiting the office because of intercurrent illness, blood glucose levels will be of little value in determining overall glycemic control, since illness generally alters glucose tolerance. Also, some patients become more conscientious about following prescribed therapy just before office visits, in which case the random plasma glucose level may be misleadingly low. For these reasons, plasma or capillary blood glucose levels should be supplemented at regular intervals with an assay for glycated hemoglobin.

Glycated Hemoglobin Concentration

Glycated hemoglobin is expressed as a percentage, i.e., the fraction of total hemoglobin that has glucose attached is glycated. Depending on the assay method and laboratory used, the test may be called glycohemoglobin, glycated hemoglobin, glycosylated hemoglobin, hemoglobin A_1, or hemoglobin A_{1c}. Although the different measurements all have different normal ranges, the results of all assay methods, when properly performed, correlate closely with each other. Efforts are underway to standardize these methods worldwide, and in the U.S., almost all assays measure A1C and are standardized to the DCCT assay. These tests are generally referred to as A1C with a normal range of 4–6%.

A glycated hemoglobin concentration may be used to assess the effects of changes in therapy made 4–12 weeks earlier. It should not be used to determine the need for short-term changes in treatment. Blood glucose levels, generally from SMBG, are still the best means by which hour-to-hour and day-to-day changes in insulin management can be determined. However, health care providers have learned not to rely solely on SMBG results because the measurements are subject to errors in technique and the records are subject to errors of omission and commission.

Certain conditions and interfering substances affect glycohemoglobin results, depending on the assay method used. Any condition that increases erythrocyte turnover, e.g., bleeding, pregnancy, or hemolysis, will spuriously lower glycohemoglobin concentration in all assays. In addition, hemoglobinopathies, e.g., sickle cell trait or disease or hemoglobin C or D, will falsely lower glycohemoglobin results when hemoglobins are separated by nonspecific methods based on charge, solubility, and size. Other conditions, e.g., uremia, high concentrations of fetal hemoglobin (HbF), high aspirin doses (usually >10 g/day), or high concentrations of ethanol, may falsely increase glycohemoglobin levels. These artifacts do not occur in all methods, and specific reference to the manufacturer's package insert for the test assay used is the best guide to a particular assay's performance in various clinical situations. A recent publication has suggested that the relationship between average blood glucose and A1C levels may be different in different ethnic populations by as much as 0.5%. However, the international A1C-Derived Average Glucose Study did not verify this. The impact of these findings is uncertain, and it is still recommended that all individuals be targeted to an A1C of <7%.

However, although the glycohemoglobin assay does reflect glycemic control over a period of 2–3 months, the result is time-weighted in that the level of glycemic control over the past month is a much greater determinant of the result than the previous months. Therefore, the glycohemoglobin test is fairly useful in assessing trends in response to therapy over a period as short as a month.

In general, well-controlled patients with type 2 diabetes and stable courses of treatment who perform home glucose monitoring should have their glycohemoglobin determined at least twice a year. More frequent monitoring of glycohemoglobin should be very useful in assessing the response to therapy in patients with unstable courses of treatment or changes in therapy and in patients on insulin therapy or those failing to achieve glycemic control goals.

SELF-MONITORING

Between office visits, the patient can assess the degree of metabolic control by performing SMBG and keeping a record of test results.

Blood Glucose Monitoring

With the advent of SMBG and the availability of multiple pharmaceutical classes of drugs that attack the pathophysiology of diabetes in different areas, near-normal glucose levels have become a realistic goal for many patients with diabetes. Although in clinical trials SMBG has not been demonstrated to change outcomes in type 2 diabetes management when evaluated in isolation, diabetes self-management has been shown to help reduce complications (e.g., the DIGAMI and Kumamoto studies). In all of these, SMBG was an integral part of the process, suggesting that SMBG is at least a component of effective therapy. SMBG, when combined with robust patient education, actively involves patients in the treatment process by allowing the patient to make adjustments in diet, exercise, and medication to achieve mutually agreed-upon targets. In the absence of periodic SMBG, it is almost impossible for patients to assess their response to the many activities that the health care team asks them to perform (e.g., nutritional changes, increased physical activity, and taking medications as prescribed). SMBG is an extraordinarily valuable tool in the education process to help ensure patient commitment to the therapeutic plan.

It is critical that patients have a well established concrete plan for action based on the results they obtain. Unfortunately, many patients faithfully perform frequent SMBG, record the results as instructed, and only discuss them with their health care team at visits, despite the fact that their control is inadequate. Unless SMBG results are within agreed-upon targets, they should be communicated and reviewed at least monthly with a member of the health care team by phone, fax, mail, e-mail, or an interim visit to trigger changes in therapy as the need arises.

SMBG is particularly recommended for all patients on insulin or sulfonylureas, as it allows for the identification of minimal and/or asymptomatic episodes of hypoglycemia. It is well recognized that recurrent mild or asymptomatic hypoglycemia is a very strong risk factor for severe hypoglycemia. Although severe hypoglycemia is relatively rare in type 2 diabetes, it can have devastating consequences, such as trauma as a result of confusion or loss of consciousness. It is also commonly accepted that mild or unrecognized hypoglycemia is part of the reason patients treated with insulin and a sulfonylurea have a proclivity for weight gain. Therefore, it is essential to have patients critically assess the nature of any "hypoglycemic" symptoms that occur during the day. Many patients are fearful or over-concerned about hypoglycemia and routinely consume extra calories when they are hungry, sweaty, nervous, or upset because they believe that they are hypoglycemic. Monitoring generally documents that most symptoms in patients with type 2 diabetes are not related to hypoglycemia and should not be treated with food.

SMBG may be useful for patients with very early type 2 diabetes treated with lifestyle management (nutrition and activity), since it allows for day-to-day determination of how adequate their efforts are. Furthermore, it gives patients the opportunity to assess glycemic excursions and contact the health care team early, if necessary, with deteriorations in glycemic control during periods of stress, such as those caused by infection or trauma.

Timing of SMBG will vary depending on the diabetes therapy. Useful times to monitor include before meals and bedtime (to assess the risk of hypoglycemia), 1–2 h after meals (to assess the maximal excursion in glucose during the day), in the middle of the sleep cycle (to assess whether there is any nocturnal hypoglycemia, which can often be asymptomatic), and when experiencing symptoms (such as "hypoglycemic spells" or illness). It is important that patients not get into the rut of only checking at one particular time of day unless they are meeting glycemic targets. There are rare individuals in whom only a certain time of day is associated with abnormal results, and in those, more focused monitoring at that time of day may be appropriate. For some patients, their highest blood glucose of the day will be the fasting glucose level or 1–2 h after breakfast. For others, their highest level will be at another time of day depending on eating habits and activity.

Likewise, there are significant numbers of patients who have near-normal levels of premeal glucose who have substantial hyperglycemic responses to meals, particularly in the context of low-fat meal plans. Both in the setting of gestational diabetes and in well-controlled type 2 diabetes, 1-h postprandial capillary blood glucose levels have correlated more strongly with glycohemoglobin than fasting or premeal glucose levels. Patients with near-normal 1-h postprandial glucose levels clearly have excellent overall glucose control.

Some clinicians have patients concentrate on premeal glucose levels if the results are generally in the high 100s or more. Once the premeal glucose levels reach the middle to low 100s, the patients switch to targeting 1- to 2-h postprandial glucose levels, since that amplifies the effects of lifestyle issues on glycemia and allows patients to identify how moderate changes in meal plan, activity, and medications have a significant impact on glycemic control. Targeting therapy to SMBG results at just one time of day could leave the patient with a less than ideal overall response to therapy.

The frequency of SMBG needs to be matched to individual patient needs and treatment. Most clinicians ask patients on hypoglycemic agents to monitor at least once a day, varying before meals, bedtime, and mid-sleep, as well as when they have hypoglycemic symptoms. Some ask insulin-treated patients to monitor much more frequently (four or more times a day). In the subset of patients who achieve stable blood glucose levels, it may be appropriate to decrease the frequency of SMBG to a few times a week, again generally concentrating on postprandial glucose levels on non-insulin therapies. It is critical that SMBG be frequent enough that the patient and provider have a good understanding of both the adequacy of the treatment regimen and the stability of glycemic control.

There is now a wide assortment of meters available with many different features that may be very important to individual patients. The meters come in a wide variety of shapes and sizes, from the size of a pen to a card to a small box. Most have some memory for previous results, and some have sophisticated features that allow the user to record medication doses and symptoms.

Some meters use significantly smaller sample volumes than others, which may be an advantage for patients who have difficulty obtaining an adequate drop. Newer meters allow sampling from alternate sites, such as the forearm. This can be very helpful to patients who have in the past used fingertips exclusively for monitoring and have scarring and pain with fingertip sampling. Some devices allow the user to wipe on blood and/or redose the strip if an inadequate volume of blood is applied to the strip initially. As a result, some meters are clearly much easier to use than others, especially for patients with a wide assortment of physical or cognitive impairments. Several can be adapted to voice synthesizers that provide audio output of results. The use of an automated lancing device for fingersticks is recommended. Several models are available: some more suited to children, those who frequently monitor, or the squeamish.

The bulk of the expense of SMBG is in the strips. It is generally possible for most patients to get a meter heavily discounted or for free. The role of the diabetes educator in helping patients determine which meter meets their needs and the role of vendors in minimizing the financial repercussions of SMBG are critical in making this technique as widely and appropriately applied as possible.

Urine Ketone Determinations

Patients with type 2 diabetes rarely have ketosis. However, some experts recommend home ketone testing in the presence of serious illness. Positive nonfasting urine ketones in a patient with type 2 diabetes are a worrisome finding that requires further evaluation.

Patient Records

The patient should be encouraged to keep a record of SMBG in tabular form, so glycemic levels at various times of the day can be scanned visually with ease. Some meters contain memories that can be downloaded into a computer to produce such glucose logs. Generally, writing down glucose levels is still preferable because it allows patients to more frequently critically assess the pattern of glucose levels over time. On a long-term basis, the burden of keeping detailed logs of glucose monitoring, food intake, doses of diabetes medications, activity, symptoms (physical as well as emotional, including their circumstance and treatment), and the relative timing of all these parameters is generally more than most patients are willing to accept. Used intermittently, these kinds of records are invaluable in assessing how various lifestyle issues and therapeutic efforts interact in determining hour-to-hour and day-to-day changes in glycemic control. They are critical in developing lifestyle plans (diet and exercise) with patients and can serve to reinforce positive behaviors and to demonstrate their beneficial outcomes.

Patient records are also helpful to the health care team because they indicate the patient's degree of interest in control and provide information necessary for development of effective therapeutic plans. Almost all patients willing to keep records should be able to achieve excellent glycemic control, since they are clearly both willing and able to make substantial efforts in their self-care behavior. Furthermore, the records are usually invaluable in providing guidance about where to concentrate efforts in trying to improve glycemic control.

BIBLIOGRAPHY

American Diabetes Association: Self-monitoring of blood glucose (Consensus Statement). *Diabetes Care* 17:81–86, 1994

American Diabetes Association: Postprandial blood glucose (Consensus Statement). *Diabetes Care* 24:775–778, 2001

American Diabetes Association: Tests of glycemia in diabetes (Position Statement). *Diabetes Care* 27:S91–S93, 2004

American Diabetes Association: Standards of medical care in diabetes: 2008 (Position Statement). *Diabetes Care* 31 (Suppl. 1):S12–S54, 2008

American Diabetes Association, European Association for the Study of Diabetes, International Federation of Clinical Chemistry and Laboratory Medicine, and the International Diabetes Federation: Consensus statement on the worldwide standardization of the hemoglobin A1C measurement. *Diabetes Care* 30:2399–2400, 2007

Dungan KM, Buse JB, Largay J, Kelly MM, Button EA, Kato S, Wittlin S: 1,5-Anhydroglucitol and postprandial hyperglycemia as measured by continuous glucose monitoring system in moderately controlled patients with diabetes. *Diabetes Care* 29:1214–1219, 2006

Dungan K, Chapman J, Braithwaite SS, Buse J: Glucose measurement: confounding issues in setting targets for inpatient management. *Diabetes Care* 30:403–409, 2007

Malmberg K, for the DIGAMI Study Group: Prospective randomized study of intensive insulin treatment on long term survival after myocardial infarction in patients with diabetes. *BMJ* 314:512–515, 1997

Ohkubo Y, Kishikawa H, Araki E, Isami S, Motoyoshi S, Kojima Y, Furuyoshi N, Shichiri M: Intensive insulin therapy prevents the progression of diabetic microvascular complications in Japanese patients with non-insulin-dependent diabetes mellitus: a randomized prospective 6-year study. *Diabetes Res Clin Prac* 28:103–117, 1995

Rohlfing CL, Wiedmeyer HM, Little RR, England JD, Tennill A, Goldstein DE: Defining the relationship between plasma glucose and HbA$_{1c}$: analysis of glucose profiles and HbA$_{1c}$ in the Diabetes Control and Complications Trial. *Diabetes Care* 25:275–278, 2002

Sacks DB, Bruns DE, Goldstein DE, MacLaren NK, McDonald JM, Parrott M: Guidelines and recommendations for laboratory analysis in the diagnosis and management of diabetes mellitus. *Diabetes Care* 25:750–786, 2002

Welschen LM, Bloemendal E, Nijpels G, Dekker JM, Heine RJ, Stalman WA, Bouter LM: Self-monitoring of blood glucose in patients with type 2 diabetes who are not using insulin: a systematic review. *Diabetes Care* 28:1510–1517, 2005

Special Therapeutic Situations

Highlights
Special Therapeutic Situations

DIABETES IN PREGNANCY

■ Glycemic control at the time of conception and throughout pregnancy is critical. Consensus on specific glycemic targets has not been achieved, but an A1C as near to normal as possible without significant hypoglycemia is recommended.

■ Insulin should be used in all pregnant patients with preexisting diabetes who fail dietary management.

■ Care for the pregnant diabetic woman should utilize a team with experience in the care of this high-risk group.

DIABETES IN YOUTH

■ Obese, inactive youth with a strong family history of type 2 diabetes are at high risk for type 2 diabetes.

■ The presence of ketoacidosis does not rule out the presence of type 2 diabetes in children.

■ Metformin is the only approved oral medication for type 2 diabetes in children.

■ Insulin should be used in children who have metabolic decompensation or who do not achieve adequate control with diet, exercise, or metformin therapy.

■ Young people with type 2 diabetes have a high risk for cardiovascular disease and should be treated aggressively for hypertension, dyslipidemia, and nephropathy.

DIABETES IN HOSPITALIZED AND CRITICALLY ILL PATIENTS

■ Intravenous insulin decreases mortality in diabetic individuals in the intensive care unit and in persons who have suffered a myocardial infarction.

■ Care of the critically ill type 2 diabetic patient should be provided through a collaboration of nursing, nutrition, and pharmacy, as well as the medical staff and patient. Institutional protocols should be developed and staff trained to allow strict glycemic control.

■ Goals of therapy in hospitalized patients should be:

Critically ill patients: as close to 110 mg/dl (post-surgical) as possible and generally <140 mg/dl

Non-critically ill patients on general medicine and surgical units, glycemic goals are less definite:

- Preprandial: <126 mg/dl
- Peak postprandial and all random glucose levels: <180–200 mg/dl

MAJOR ACUTE COMPLICATIONS

■ The major acute complications of diabetes include metabolic problems and infection.

■ The two metabolic problems of most concern in patients with type 2 diabetes are hyperosmolar hyperglycemic state and hypoglycemia in patients treated with insulin or insulin secretagogues. Diabetic ketoacidosis may occur occasionally in patients with type 2 diabetes under severe stress (including severe infection).

■ The four major clinical features of hyperosmolar hyperglycemic state are:

- severe hyperglycemia
- absence of or slight ketosis
- plasma or serum hyperosmolality
- profound dehydration

■ Hypoglycemia can be precipitated by:

- decreased food intake
- intensive exercise
- alcohol and other drugs in combination with exogenous insulin, sulfonylureas and meglitinides

■ Hypoglycemia should be suspected in a patient who presents with manifestations of altered mental and/or neurologic function as well as adrenergic responses. The diagnosis is confirmed by a plasma glucose level <60 mg/dl (<3.3 mmol/l).

■ If the patient is conscious, hypoglycemia should be treated by oral ingestion of some form of sugar. In the unconscious patient, parenteral glucagon or intravenous glucose may be necessary.

Special Therapeutic Situations

Diabetes can cause unique clinical complications for both the pregnant patient and her baby. The infant of a mother with preexisting diabetes has an increased risk of death, prematurity, and morbidity (congenital defects, macrosomia and related delivery disorders, hypoglycemia, hypocalcemia, hyperbilirubinemia, and respiratory distress syndrome). The mother with preexisting diabetes faces the risk of accelerating microvascular complications involving the kidneys and eyes, particularly if complications and hypertension are present. Tight glucose control is essential from conception through delivery to reduce the risks of both maternal and neonatal complications.

A large proportion of women with type 2 diabetes are obese and have insulin resistance and associated metabolic disorders. This can lead to additional complications, including preeclampsia, placental insufficiency, cardiac dysfunction, sleep apnea, and nonalcoholic fatty liver disease. Recommendations for weight gain during pregnancy in obese individuals are currently under review but should be limited at least to the lower limits of general guidelines, and physical activity should be encouraged.

In a patient with preexisting diabetes, pregnancy should be planned so that conception occurs when the patient has near-normal fasting, preprandial, and postprandial plasma glucose levels and A1C values within the goal range. After conception, treatment should not only continue to achieve glycemic goals, but also meet the nutritional requirements of the fetus. Although several recent studies have suggested that glyburide is relatively safe and effective for treating gestational diabetes, it has not been studied in the setting of type 2 diabetes and pregnancy. Given the expected increase in insulin requirements during pregnancy, it is almost a certainty that patients with preexisting diabetes would fail to maintain glycemic goals on these oral agents during pregnancy. It is currently recommended that oral diabetes medications, with the possible exception of metformin, be stopped before conception. Insulin therapy should be initiated and titrated to achieve glycemic goals before conception.

The physician should inform the patient of the risks to her and the baby. Because the risks of pregnancy in the setting of preexisting diabetes are increased for both mother and fetus/newborn and the treatment program (multiple injections of insulin or use of the insulin pump and euglycemic regulation) is complex, the care of a pregnant woman with diabetes should involve appropriate specialists. Consultation with a physician skilled in the care of pregnant women with preexisting diabetes should be sought before conception or as soon as pregnancy is diagnosed to effect normalization of blood glucose levels. Finally, it is important to recognize that offspring of obese insulin-resistant woman are at an increased risk for childhood obesity and early onset of metabolic disorders associated with obesity, including cardiovascular risk factors and type 2 diabetes.

Glycemic control in diabetic women during pregnancy should try to achieve near-normal glucose levels and A1C as close to normal as possible without causing undue risk from hypoglycemia.

The care of a pregnant woman with diabetes is best accomplished by an experienced health care team. The team must be completely familiar with proper management of the patient and her fetus/newborn during pregnancy, just before and during delivery, and immediately after delivery. The same vigorous attention to glycemic regulation and proper management of the patient and her fetus/newborn must be given to the individual who develops gestational diabetes during the second or third trimester.

BIBLIOGRAPHY

Catalano PM: Management of obesity in pregnancy. *Obstet Gynecol* 109:419–433, 2007

Crowther CA, Hiller JE, Moss JR, McPhee AJ, Jeffries WS, Robinson JS, Australian Carbohydrate Intolerance Study in Pregnant Women (ACHOIS) Trial Group: Effect of treatment of gestational diabetes mellitus on pregnancy outcomes. *N Engl J Med* 352:2477–2486, 2005

Kitzmiller JL, et al.: *Preexisting Diabetes and Pregnancy.* Alexandria, VA, American Diabetes Association, 2008

The pathophysiology of type 2 diabetes in young individuals is likely very similar to that seen in adults, with obesity and physical inactivity as primary inciting factors. Given the direct relationship between weight gain and the risk for diabetes, it is not surprising that the recent rise in obesity in young people is paralleled by an increase in the number of cases of type 2 diabetes. At least 15% of adolescents are defined as overweight and the incidence is rising, especially among minority children. In some communities, obesity rates are 33–50% and the incidence of type 2 diabetes is surpassing type 1 diabetes as the primary cause of diabetes in children. The increase in obesity in youth is related to both decreases in physical activity and consumption of food with high caloric density. In the U.S., 27% of high school boys and 43% of high school girls are estimated to have an insufficient amount of physical activity. Leisure-time physical activity decreases with age and is directly related to time spent viewing television. Studies have also demonstrated a correlation between television viewing and consumption of high-energy foods, further contributing to obesity.

DIFFERENTIATION OF TYPE 1 AND TYPE 2 DIABETES IN YOUTH

In the adolescent, type 2 diabetes can be differentiated from type 1 diabetes by the presence of significant obesity, the absence of islet cell antibodies, and normal or elevated fasting C-peptide levels. In many instances, there will be acanthosis nigricans and there is usually a significant family history of type 2 diabetes. The young person with type 2 diabetes typically does not present with significant weight loss but may have ketonuria and even ketoacidosis. It has been suggested that the onset of puberty in obese children may be an inciting event for the development of diabetes in this susceptible population.

SCREENING FOR TYPE 2 DIABETES IN YOUTH

A significant rise in the incidence of type 2 diabetes in children has prompted a reassessment of screening criteria for this group. The American Diabetes Association and the American Academy of Pediatrics have promulgated criteria for screening in the pediatric population (Table 4.1). It recommends testing at >10 years of age or at the onset of puberty in children with a BMI >85th percentile, with a first- or second-degree relative having diabetes, and in an at-risk racial/ethnic group, particularly with signs of insulin resistance such as acanthosis nigricans, hypertension, polycystic ovarian syndrome (PCOS), or dyslipidemia. Fasting plasma glucose is the preferred screening modality, although a 2-h glucose tolerance test can be used.

The majority of children with type 2 diabetes do not have underlying diseases that cause obesity. It is therefore not routinely recommended that screening for other causes be undertaken unless there is clinical evidence for diseases such as hypothyroidism or Cushing's disease. Serum triglyceride levels are often elevated in obese children, and it is recommended that these children have a fasting lipid panel performed. Liver function tests should be obtained to detect asymptomatic nonalcoholic fatty liver. Children with persistent liver function tests greater than twofold normal should be evaluated for non-metabolic causes of liver disease (viral hepatitis, Wilson disease, autoimmune hepatitis, and α_1-antitrypsin deficiency).

Table 4.1 Criteria for Screening the Pediatric Population

Criteria
- Overweight (BMI >85th percentile for age and sex, weight for height >85th percentile, or weight >120% of ideal for height)

Plus any two of the following risk factors:
- Family history of type 2 diabetes in first- or second-degree relative
- Race/ethnicity (e.g., Native American, African American, Latino, Asian American, and Pacific Islander)
- Signs of insulin resistance or conditions associated with insulin resistance (e.g., acanthosis nigricans, hypertension, dyslipidemia, or PCOS)
- Maternal history of diabetes or gestational diabetes

Age of initiation: age 10 years or at onset of puberty, if puberty occurs at a younger age

Frequency: every 2 years
Test: Fasting plasma glucose preferred

From the American Diabetes Association, 2008.

TREATING TYPE 2 DIABETES IN YOUTH

The approach to treatment of pediatric type 2 diabetes is complicated by the fact that there are currently few data comparing the relative efficacies of diet, exercise, insulin, and other drug therapies in this population. However, given the early onset of type 2 diabetes, aggressive therapies are required because of the longer diabetes duration and subsequent risk for macrovascular and microvascular complications. An aggressive intervention directed toward weight loss, including dietary restriction and exercise, along with an educational plan that includes the family caregivers, is an essential part of the therapeutic plan. Especially important is education of the patient and family, with the goal of decreasing intake of caloric-dense foods, such as saturated fats and candy. In addition, a family-based progressive increase in physical activity and reduction of sedentary activities (e.g., video games) should be emphasized. Currently, two medications, orlistat and sibutramine, are approved in the United States for weight management in adolescents. These may be useful in conjunction with lifestyle modification to enhance weight loss. In addition, bariatric surgery may be considered in morbidly obese children who have failed medical and pharmacologic treatment for obesity. This latter option should be approached with caution, since few long-term outcome studies have been performed in adolescents who have undergone these procedures.

Goals of treatment in this population include the achievement of near-normal glycemic control (A1C at least <7% or as close to normal as possible without hypoglycemia) to reduce risk for microvascular and macrovascular complications.

Exogenous insulin has traditionally been used to treat childhood diabetes, and this should be instituted in individuals with significant elevations of glucose and in anyone demonstrating ketosis. Early administration of insulin may increase compliance, perhaps by conveying a message as to the significance of the disease. Insulin therapy is associated with weight gain, and early institution of medical nutrition therapy is imperative. Once glucose control is established, it may be possible to transition the patient to oral medications.

While many oral agents are available to treat type 2 diabetes in adults and all have been used in children, metformin is the only oral drug approved by the Food and Drug Administration to treat type 2 diabetes in children. Metformin can decrease A1C by ~1% in this population. Sulfonylureas are effective in adults but are associated with hypoglycemia and weight gain and therefore should not be used as first-line agents. Whereas theoretically attractive from their insulin-sensitizing effect, the glitazone class of medication has not been extensively studied in the pediatric population. Recent concerns regarding an increased risk of bone fracture in postmenopausal women treated with glitazones, as well as conflicting data on their cardiovascular impact, increase concern for long-term use in pediatric populations.

As in adults, dyslipidemia and hypertension should be treated aggressively and prevention or cessation of smoking is a critical component of care. Screening and treatment with angiotensin-converting enzyme inhibitors for microalbuminuria should be part of the treatment plan. In general, aspirin should be avoided until age 21 because of concerns about Reye's Syndrome in children. Goals for therapy are outlined in Table 4.2. Dietary lipid management is the initial treatment imperative, with addition of a statin if indicated in older children.

Table 4.2 Recommendations for Monitoring Blood Pressure and Lipid Levels in Youth

Blood Pressure
Normal blood pressure levels for age, sex, and height; appropriate methods for measurement; and treatment recommendations are available at www.nhlbi.nih.gov/health/prof/heart/hbp/hbp_ped.pdf.

An average systolic or diastolic blood pressure should be measured on at least three separate days. A pressure greater than the 95th percentile for age, sex, and height is considered abnormal.

Angiotensin-converting enzyme inhibitors are preferred in children with microalbuminuria.

Lipids
A lipid profile should be obtained after glucose levels are controlled and should be monitored at 3- to 5-year intervals if normal.

Treatment goals are:
- LDL cholesterol <100 mg/dl
- HDL cholesterol >35 mg/dl
- Triglycerides <150 mg/dl

If the LDL cholesterol level is >100 mg/dl, an exercise and diet should be prescribed. If goals are not reached after 6 months, consider statin therapy after the age of 10 for patients with an LDL cholesterol level of 130–159 mg/dl. Patients with an LDL cholesterol level >160 mg/dl should have therapy initiated. Statins appear to be safe for children, although niacin and cholestyramine are also treatment options.

BIBLIOGRAPHY

American Diabetes Association: Management of dyslipidemia in children and adolescents with diabetes. *Diabetes Care* 26:2194–2197, 2003

American Diabetes Association: Standards of medical care in diabetes. *Diabetes Care* 31 (Suppl. 1):S12–S54, 2008

Aye T, Levitsky LL: Type 2 diabetes: an epidemic disease in childhood. *Curr Opin Pediatr* 15:411–415, 2003

Bloomgarden ZT: Type 2 diabetes in the young: the evolving epidemic. *Diabetes Care* 27:998–1010, 2004

Peterson K, Silverstein J, Kaufman F, Warren-Boulton E: Management of type 2 diabetes in youth: an update. *Am Fam Physician* 76:658–664, 2007

Pinhas-Hamiel O, Zeitler P: Acute and chronic complications of type 2 diabetes mellitus in children and adolescents. *Lancet* 369:1823–1831, 2007

Spear BA, Barlow SE, Ervin C, Ludwig DS, Saelens BE, Schetzina KE, Taveras EM: Recommendations for treatment of child and adolescent overweight and obesity. *Pediatrics* 120 (Suppl. 4):S254–S288, 2007

DIABETES IN HOSPITALIZED AND CRITICALLY ILL PATIENTS

Numerous observational studies as well as randomized prospective trials using intravenous insulin therapy have revolutionized our thinking about postoperative and inpatient care of diabetes and hyperglycemia by demonstrating that intensive insulin treatment of critically ill hospitalized patients can reduce mortality and improve hospital outcomes. Patients had reduced mortality when presenting with acute myocardial infarction and randomized to intravenous infusion of insulin (containing potassium chloride) titrated to achieve glucose levels of 126–180 mg/dl followed by multiple daily injections for outpatient blood glucose control. A second report demonstrated that intravenous insulin infusion in the surgical intensive care unit (ICU) to achieve target glucose of 80–110 mg/dl reduced the risk of in-hospital mortality in general, with a specific benefit on reducing the risk associated with infectious complications of prolonged ICU treatment. A similar intervention for medical ICU patients showed reduced morbidity but no difference in mortality and showed higher hypoglycemia rates. Numerous professional organizations now suggest that the treatment of diabetes and hyperglycemia in the hospital should target plasma glucose levels approaching normoglycemia:

- Critically ill patients: as close to 110 mg/dl (post-surgical) as possible and generally <140 mg/dl
- Non-critically ill patients on general medicine and surgical units, glycemic goals are less definite:
  - Preprandial: <126 mg/dl
  - Peak postprandial and all random glucose levels: <180–200 mg/dl

Achieving such levels of glycemic control in the hectic inpatient environment does challenge patients, health care providers, and health care systems and requires the collaboration of nursing, nutrition, and pharmacy as well as the medical staff and patient. Institutional protocols should be developed and staff trained to allow these levels of control to be achieved. Preprinted order sets facilitate adherence to protocols, and numerous examples are now available in the literature.

Most authorities advocate intravenous infusion of insulin instead of subcutaneous administration in the OR and the ICU. To the extent that intravenous administration can be used elsewhere in the health care system, it makes it possible to carefully control the amount of insulin delivered based on frequent measurement of blood glucose and changes in diet, medication, and severity of illness.

Unless the surgical condition is an emergency, the patient should be allowed sufficient time to achieve acceptable control of hyperglycemia before surgery. If possible, the patient should have a complete evaluation of metabolic state and thorough assessment of diabetic complications, including renal and cardiovascular disease, before surgery.

It is now possible for a patient with diabetes to undergo surgical operations with little more than normal risk, unless the operation is done under emergency conditions that do not allow complete evaluation and preparation of the patient.

The objectives of management before, during, and after surgery are to prevent hypoglycemia, which can lead to coma, and to prevent excessive hyperglycemia and ketoacidosis, which can complicate postoperative care by increasing the risk of major infections, thrombosis, dehydration, excessive protein loss, and electrolyte imbalance. To accomplish these ends, the anesthetic technique (regional or general) and the anesthetic agent should disrupt metabolic control as little as possible. Special attention should be given to maintaining proper fluid and electrolyte balance and blood glucose levels. Patients with diabetes who have been treated with diet or oral agents may need insulin therapy for control of hyperglycemia during the acute stress period of a major surgical procedure. Most oral agents may need to be replaced by insulin during a hospital stay. The suggested components of successful insulin treatment include basal (as intermediate- or long-acting insulin), bolus, and correction (both as short- or rapid-acting insulin) insulin.

To assume responsibility for the management of patients with type 2 diabetes during hospital stays, the clinician must be adept at principles and specific techniques in the management of hospital hyperglycemia. Major principles governing such management are presented in Table 4.3.

Table 4.3 Major Principles Governing Management of Patients with Diabetes During Hospitalization

- Metabolic control is associated with improved hospital outcomes. Target plasma glucose levels on general floors are <110 mg/dl (<126 mg/dl fasting) preprandial and <180–200 mg/dl peak postprandial or random.

- Intensive insulin therapy with intravenous insulin, with the goal of maintaining blood glucose of 80–110 mg/dl in surgical patients and generally <140 mg/dl in other patients, reduces morbidity and mortality among critically ill patients.

- Intravenous insulin infusion is safe and effective for achieving metabolic control during major surgery, hemodynamic instability, and NPO status.

- Intravenous insulin infusion is safe and effective for patients who have poorly controlled diabetes and widely fluctuating blood glucose levels or who are insulin deficient or severely insulin resistant.

- Intravenous insulin infusion, followed by multi-dose subcutaneous insulin therapy, improves survival in diabetic patients after myocardial infarction.

- For insulin-deficient patients, despite reductions or the absence of caloric intake, basal insulin must be provided to prevent diabetic ketoacidosis.

- Use of scheduled insulin provided as basal, bolus, and correctional therapy improves blood glucose control compared with sliding-scale insulin coverage alone.

- For patients who are alert and demonstrate accurate insulin self-administration and glucose monitoring, insulin self-management should be allowed as an adjunct to standard nurse-delivered diabetes management.

- Patients with no prior history of diabetes who are found to have hyperglycemia (random [fasting] blood glucose >126 mg/dl or 6.9 mmol/l) during hospitalization should have follow-up testing for diabetes within 1 month of hospital discharge.

- Establishing a multidisciplinary team that sets and implements institutional guidelines, protocols, and standardized order sets for the hospital results in reduced hypoglycemic and hyperglycemic events.

- Diabetes education, medical nutrition therapy, and timely diabetes-specific discharge planning are essential components of hospital-based diabetes care.

From Clement et al., 2004.

BIBLIOGRAPHY

Clement S, Braithwaite SS, Magee MF, Ahmann A, Smith EP, Schafer RG, Hirsch IB: Management of diabetes and hyperglycemia in hospitals. *Diabetes Care* 27:553–591, 2004

Pittas AG, Siegel RD, Lau J: Insulin therapy and in-hospital mortality in critically ill patients: systematic review and meta-analysis of randomized controlled trials. *JPEN J Parenter Enteral Nutr* 30:164–172, 2006

MAJOR ACUTE COMPLICATIONS

In this section, the acute metabolic complications of diabetes, including the hyperosmolar hyperglycemic state and hypoglycemia and their management, are reviewed. Patients with type 2 diabetes are often treated with numerous medications, including hypoglycemic, antihypertensive, and hypolipidemic drugs, to treat their diabetes and common coexistent disorders. The adverse effects of these medications and their interactions are also reviewed.

The major acute complications of diabetes include metabolic problems and infection. The two metabolic problems of most concern in patients with type 2 diabetes are hyperosmolar hyperglycemic nonketotic syndrome and hypoglycemia.

HYPEROSMOLAR HYPERGLYCEMIC STATE

Of all diabetic comas, hyperosmolar hyperglycemic state (HHS) is the most common in older patients with type 2 diabetes. When this condition occurs, it can be life-threatening. HHS sometimes occurs in people with undiagnosed diabetes and in those with diagnosed diabetes after long periods of uncontrolled hyperglycemia.

Precipitating causes

There is almost always a precipitating factor (Table 4.4). Precipitating events include the use of drugs as well as other acute and chronic diseases (particularly infection) that increase glucose levels. Abnormal thirst sensation or limited access to water also facilitate development of this syndrome.

Table 4.4 Factors Associated with the Hyperosmolar Hyperglycemic State

Therapeutic Agents	Therapeutic Procedures	Chronic Diseases	Acute Situations
Glucocorticoids	Peritoneal dialysis	Renal disease	Infection
Diuretics	Hemodialysis	Heart disease	Diabetic gangrene
Diphenylhydantoin	Hyperosmolar alimentation	Hypertension	Urinary tract infection
α-Aderenergic-blocking agents	Surgical stress	Dementia	Septicemia
Diazoxide		Old stroke	Extensive burns
L-Asparaginase		Alcoholism	Gastrointestinal hemorrhage
Immunosuppressive agents		Psychiatric loss of thirst	Cerebrovascular accident
			Myocardial infarction
			Pancreatitis

Adapted from Garcia de los Rio, 1982, and Podolsky, 1981.

Clinical presentation

There are four major clinical features of HHS:

1. Severe hyperglycemia (blood glucose >600 mg/dl [>33.3 mmol/l] and generally between 1,000 and 2,000 mg/dl [55.5–111.1 mmol/l])
2. Absence of or slight ketosis
3. Plasma or serum hyperosmolality (>340 mOsm/kg)
4. Profound dehydration

Typically, the patient develops excessive thirst, altered sensorium (coma or confusion), and physical signs of severe dehydration.

Treatment

The precipitating event should be determined and corrected as soon as possible, and lifesaving measures should be used immediately. Dehydration, hyperglycemia, electrolyte abnormalities, and the hyperosmolar condition should be corrected with use of appropriate fluids, insulin, and potassium.

HYPOGLYCEMIA

This metabolic problem is a greater problem and is more frequent in patients with type 1 diabetes than in patients with type 2 diabetes. However, it certainly can develop in patients with type 2 diabetes treated with insulin or insulin secretagogues.

Precipitating causes

Hypoglycemia results when there is an imbalance between food intake and the appropriate dosage of drug therapy (i.e., sulfonylureas, meglitinides, insulin, or a combination of these drugs). Exercise, intake of alcohol or other drugs, or decreased liver or kidney function can precipitate or exacerbate this imbalance.

Clinical presentation

Hypoglycemia should be suspected in a patient who presents with symptoms indicative of altered mental and/or neurological function (changes in sensorium and behavior, coma, or seizure), as well as adrenergic responses (tachycardia, palpitations, increased sweating, and hunger). The diagnosis is confirmed if a plasma glucose level of <60 mg/dl (<3.3 mmol/l) is found when the patient is symptomatic.

Treatment

The objective of treatment is to restore the plasma glucose level to normal. When the patient is conscious and cooperative, ingestion of some form of glucose by mouth (e.g., fruit juice, sugar cubes, glucose tablets, or a solution equivalent to 15–20 g carbohydrate) is usually followed by rapid relief of symptoms. In the unconscious or uncooperative patient, parenteral glucagon or intravenous glucose (50 ml 50% dextrose or glucose followed by 5% or 10% dextrose drip) should be given. In the setting of hypoglycemia secondary to sulfonylureas, hypoglycemia may be prolonged, and patients should be observed for at least 12–24 h.

INFECTION

The rapid diagnosis and treatment of infection in a patient with diabetes is absolutely necessary because infection is a leading cause of metabolic abnormalities leading to diabetic coma. The more common infections seen in patients with diabetes and some critical comments about them are presented in Table 4.5.

Table 4.5 Infections That Are Common or Special to Patients with Diabetes

Type of Infection	Comment
Cutaneous furunculosis and carbuncles	For reasons not clear, patients with diabetes may be prone to recurrent furunculosis and carbuncles. Unless vascular insufficiency is present, warm compresses may be used for treatment.
Vulvovaginitis (less frequently scrotal infections)	*Candida* skin infection commonly occurs in warm, moist areas, particularly in the region of the genitalia (also on the inner thighs and under the breasts). This is particularly common in people with type 2 diabetes who are overweight or who have been taking antibiotics. These infections can cause extreme discomfort to the patient and result in breakdown of skin, which may allow entry of more virulent organisms. Good glycemic control and local supportive antifungal treatment usually will resolve the problem.
Cellulitis, alone or in combination with lower-extremity vascular ulcers	To prevent the spread of infection to bone and the necessity of amputation, treatment of infected ulcers and surrounding cellulitis must be aggressive. Antibiotics effective against bacteria recovered from the site (both aerobes and anaerobes should be expected), as well as surgical debridement and drainage, should be used.
Urinary tract	Asymptomatic bacteriuria occurs in up to 20% of patients with diabetes; some suggest that it be treated. Certainly a patient with neurogenic bladder is susceptible to urinary tract infection and sepsis. Treatment is mandatory in patients with pyelonephritis. Patients with serious urinary tract infections should be hospitalized, the offending pathogens identified, and appropriate susceptibility tests performed.
Ear	Malignant external otitis is relatively rare, but when it occurs, it is most often seen in elderly patients with chronically draining ear and sudden onset of severe pain. *Pseudomonas aeruginosa* is the usual pathogenic organism. This condition is fatal in ~50% of cases. Immediate treatment should include appropriate antibiotic therapy and surgical debridement when indicated.

Adapted from Casey, 1984.

BIBLIOGRAPHY

Casey JI: Host defense and infections in diabetes mellitus. In *Ellenberg and Rifkin's Diabetes Mellitus: Therapy and Practice.* 3rd ed. Ellenberg M, Rifkin H, Eds. New York, NY, Elsevier Science, 1984

Garcia de los Rio M: Nonketotic hyperosmolar coma. In *World Book of Diabetes Practice 1982.* Krall LP, Alberti KGMM, Eds. Amsterdam, the Netherlands, Excerpta Medica, 1982, p. 96–99

Podolsky S: Hyperosmolar nonketotic coma. In *Diabetes Mellitus.* Vol. V. Rifkin H, Raskin P, Eds. Bowie, MD, Brady, 1981

Detection and Treatment of Chronic Complications

Highlights
Detection and Treatment
of Chronic Complications

■ In the U.S., kidney failure, blindness, amputations, and cardiovascular disease (CVD) resulting from diabetes markedly reduce quality and length of life and cost more than $170 billion annually.

■ Success in the prevention and treatment of diabetes-related complications is only achieved with a motivated multidisciplinary approach in which communication and collaborative efforts are optimized.

CARDIOVASCULAR DISEASE

■ The risk of myocardial infarction in a subject with diabetes is equivalent to that of a nondiabetic subject who has already suffered a myocardial infarction.

■ In type 2 diabetes, common co-existent conditions, including hypertension, dyslipidemia (decreased HDL cholesterol, increased triglycerides, and alterations in LDL cholesterol particle size and number), hypercoagulability, and obesity, are also cardiovascular risk factors.

DIABETIC RETINOPATHY

■ The risk of developing diabetic retinopathy is closely related to the duration of diabetes and the degree of antecedent hyperglycemia.

DIABETIC NEPHROPATHY

■ Diabetic nephropathy occurs in 20–40% of individuals with diabetes and is the leading cause of end-stage renal disease.

DIABETIC FOOT PROBLEMS

■ More than 50% of the nontraumatic amputations in the U.S. occur in individuals with diabetes, and it has been estimated that >50% of these amputations could have been prevented with proper care.

DIABETIC NEUROPATHY

■ The diabetic neuropathies include the polyneuropathies of the upper and lower extremities and autonomic nervous system, lumbosacral plexus neuropathies, truncal radiculopathy, upper limb mononeuropathies, and cranial neuropathy.

- Neuropathic foot ulcers are a complication of lower-extremity polyneuropathy.

- The autonomic neuropathies include gastroparesis, diabetic diarrhea/constipation, neurogenic bladder, impaired cardiovascular reflexes and orthostatic hypotension, impaired glucose counterregulation, and sexual dysfunction.

- Therapy is principally directed toward early diagnosis, prevention of foot complications, and amelioration of troubling symptoms.

Detection and Treatment of Chronic Complications

M any clinicians consider type 2 diabetes a "mild" form of diabetes compared with type 1 diabetes because, characteristically, patients have less labile glucose profiles and can often be managed satisfactorily with nutrition and exercise therapy, plus non-insulin therapies. Consequently, these patients have traditionally not been offered therapy geared to optimizing their metabolic control.

However, people with type 2 diabetes are afflicted with the same devastating litany of diabetes-specific long-term microvascular and neurological complications as patients with type 1 diabetes (Table 5.1). Several recent trials such as the U.K. Prospective Diabetes Study (UKPDS) and Kumamoto Study showed that improved glycemic control in individuals with type 2 diabetes reduces their rate of diabetic complications. In addition, type 2 diabetes generally affects an older population and is commonly accompanied by a high prevalence of cardiovascular risk factors. This combination of characteristics magnifies the risk of premature cardiac, cerebral, and peripheral vascular disease two- to sevenfold compared with the nondiabetic population.

These complications—loss of vision, renal failure requiring dialysis or transplantation, amputations, heart attacks, strokes, and premature mortality—cause immense burden to patients and belie the notion that type 2 diabetes is mild. Because of the "silent" onset of type 2 diabetes in many, up to 50% of individuals already have complications at diagnosis. Type 2 diabetes accounts for >90% of diabetes in the United States, affecting over 20 million people, and therefore is a major burden to our health care system. For example, type 2 diabetes is the single most common cause of new cases of end-stage renal disease (ESRD).

This section reviews the detection, prevention, and treatment of long-term diabetes microvascular (retinopathy, nephropathy, and neuropathy) and macrovascular (coronary, cerebrovascular, and peripheral) complications that accompany type 2 diabetes. Patient cases that illustrate proper diagnosis, prevention, and treatment of diabetic complications are presented.

RATIONALE FOR OPTIMIZING GLYCEMIC CONTROL IN TYPE 2 DIABETES

A strong association between hyperglycemia and microvascular disease risk has emerged from epidemiologic studies and then intervention studies designed to assess whether improved glucose control delays the development and progression of retinopathy, nephropathy, and neuropathy in patients with either type 1 or type 2

Table 5.1 Chronic Complications Associated with Type 2 Diabetes

Vascular Diseases

- Macrovascular
  - Accelerated coronary atherosclerosis
  - Accelerated cerebrovascular atherosclerosis
  - Accelerated peripheral vascular disease
- Microvascular
  - Retinopathy
  - Nephropathy

Neuropathy Syndromes and Outcomes

- Sensorimotor neuropathy
  - Symmetrical polyneuropathy, bilateral (lower > upper limbs)
    - Pain
    - Foot deformity
    - Ulceration
  - Mononeuropathy
  - Diabetic amyotrophy
  - Neuropathic cachexia
- Autonomic neuropathy
  - Gastroparesis
  - Diabetic diarrhea
  - Neurogenic bladder
  - Sexual dysfunction
  - Orthostatic hypotension

Mixed Vascular and Neuropathic Diseases

- Leg ulcers
- Foot ulcers

diabetes. In type 2 diabetes, evidence supporting the role of treating hyperglycemia in the reduction of diabetic microvascular complications initially emerged in the Kumamoto Study and was confirmed in the larger UKPDS. The UKPDS evaluated the effects of intensive blood glucose control (to achieve a fasting plasma glucose goal <6 mmol/l [<108 mg/dl]) with sulfonylurea, metformin, or insulin and less intensive treatment with nutrition therapy versus conventional treatment (to maintain a fasting plasma glucose goal of <15 mmol/l [<270 mg/dl] without symptoms of hyperglycemia) on the risk of microvascular and macrovascular complications in patients newly diagnosed with type 2 diabetes. Over 10 years, A1C averaged 7.0% in the intensive group compared with 7.9% in the conventionally treated group—an 11% reduction. There were no differences in A1C values among the patients randomized to either oral hypoglycemic agents or insulin therapy in the intensive treatment group. Compared with less intensive therapy, intensive therapy reduced the risk by 12% for any diabetes-related end point. Most of this benefit was due to a 25% relative risk reduction in microvascular end points, including the need for retinal photocoagulation. Moreover, achieving and maintaining A1C goals for a prolonged time period appeared to reduce the risk of subsequently developing complications, even if the glucose control deteriorated. The term "metabolic memory" has been invoked to describe this effect. These data strongly support the beneficial effects of effective antihyperglycemic therapy on the prevention of microvascular disease, regardless of the pathophysiology of the hyperglycemia.

Improved glycemic control also reduced the incidence of macrovascular complications in the UKPDS, but this was not statistically significant. There was a 16% risk reduction of myocardial infarction (MI) and sudden death, but diabetes-related mortality and all-cause mortality did not differ between the intensive and conventionally treated groups. A secondary randomization involved overweight patients with diabetes. In this substudy, patients treated with metformin, compared with the conventional group, had risk reductions of 32% for any diabetes-related end point, 42% for diabetes-related death, and 36% for all-cause mortality. There was an intermediate and statistically significant reduction when overweight patients were treated with insulin or sulfonylurea. Therefore, metformin therapy appears to decrease the risk of macrovascular disease in obese patients with type 2 diabetes. Further studies are in progress to explore optimal treatment strategies for decreasing the excess cardiovascular disease (CVD) risk in type 2 diabetes.

Good glycemic control reflected by A1C goals of <7% should therefore be reinforced and promoted at every opportunity. More stringent goals (i.e., a normal A1C <6%) should be considered in high-risk individual patients based on epidemiological observations suggesting a continuum rather than a threshold for glycemia and the risk of complications. Treatment should always be individualized, taking into consideration the patient's age and prognosis.

ACCELERATED MACROVASCULAR DISEASE

In the patient with diabetes, atherosclerosis involving the coronary, cerebrovascular, and peripheral vessels occurs at an earlier age and with greater frequency than it does in people without diabetes and is responsible for two-thirds of the mortality in adults with diabetes. Thus, the clinician should be alert for signs and symptoms of accelerated atherosclerosis among patients with diabetes.

Although many patients with diabetes experience the same symptoms of coronary, cerebral, and peripheral vascular disease as patients without diabetes, clinicians should be aware that neuropathy and other factors may alter symptoms in the patient with diabetes. At least one-third of patients with diabetes with coronary disease have no or atypical anginal symptoms, such as exertional dyspnea, rather than exertional chest pain. In addition, cerebral manifestations of hypoglycemia may mimic transient ischemic attacks, and symptoms of neuropathy may need to be distinguished from symptoms of intermittent claudication.

DIABETES AS A CARDIOVASCULAR RISK FACTOR

Studies have shown consistently that patients with diabetes have an excess of cardiovascular complications compared with patients without diabetes. In the United States, for example, those with diabetes are two- to fourfold as likely as age-matched individuals without diabetes to die from coronary artery disease, and the average annual incidence of cardiovascular sequelae is increased at least twofold in patients with diabetes. The risk of MI in a subject with diabetes is equivalent to that of a nondiabetic subject who has already suffered an MI. Most importantly, the relative risk for CVD in women with type 2 diabetes is three to four times greater than for age-matched women without diabetes. In addition, women with diabetes complicated by coronary vessel disease appear to have particularly bad outcomes, emphasizing the need for aggressive management in this population.

Type 2 diabetes is an independent risk factor for macrovascular disease. In addition, common coexistent conditions, including hypertension, dyslipidemia (decreased HDL cholesterol, increased triglycerides, and alterations in LDL cholesterol particle size and number), hypercoagulability, and obesity, are also risk factors. The pattern of obesity is important, with central fat distribution (waist circumference >40 inches in men and >35 inches in women) associated with dyslipidemia, hypertension, and increased prevalence of CVD, independent of obesity. Other risk factors demonstrated in people without diabetes, such as smoking and lack of exercise, apply as well to people with type 2 diabetes. Finally, renal failure, retinopathy, cardiac autonomic neuropathy, and microalbuminuria are additional markers of increased cardiovascular risk.

SCREENING FOR CARDIOVASCULAR DISEASE

Diagnostic testing for coronary artery disease should be considered in subjects with either typical or atypical cardiac symptoms or an abnormal resting ECG. In such patients, the pretest probability of an abnormal test is sufficiently high that a stress test with imaging procedure such as stress echocardiography or nuclear stress imaging or a cardiac catheterization is appropriate.

In terms of asymptomatic patients, older recommendations were to screen for CAD in older patients with multiple CVD risk factors. However, trials of screening in subjects with type 2 diabetes have found no association between risk factor burden and ischemia on testing. In addition, aggressive medical therapy of CVD risk factors is associated with reversal of ischemia in a high proportion of cases, and in patients with stable angina has equivalent outcomes to percutaneous intervention. In light of this growing body of evidence, a 2007 ADA consensus statement did not recommend routine CAD screening for asymptomatic patients. Rather, all patients with diabetes and moderate or high CVD risk should have aggressive medical therapy for all risk factors.

IMPORTANCE OF MODIFYING VASCULAR RISK FACTORS

Lifestyle measures, including weight reduction and exercise for overweight and obese patients with type 2 diabetes, are the most cost-effective and safest modes of therapy and should be included in all treatment regimens. Successful weight reduction will improve atherogenic lipid profiles, glucose intolerance, hypertension, and of course obesity. The National Institutes of Health–funded Look-AHEAD Trial is examining the impact of aggressive lifestyle intervention on CVD outcomes in type 2 diabetes.

Although most studies demonstrating the efficacy of reducing cardiovascular risk factors, such as hypertension and hyperlipidemia, in preventing or ameliorating CVD have been performed in populations without diabetes, evidence from several studies suggests that such interventions will similarly benefit individuals with type 2 diabetes. The cardiovascular benefits for patients with type 2 diabetes of lowering blood pressure and LDL cholesterol were documented in the UKPDS and in diabetic subgroups from several major statin trials. More recently, the Heart Protection Study demonstrated that in people with diabetes age >40 years with total cholesterol >135 mg/dl, LDL reductions of ~30% with simvastatin were associated with an ~25% reduction in coronary events, independent of baseline LDL levels, prior vascular disease, or type 1 or type 2 diabetes. Similarly, in CARDS (Coronary Artery Diabetes Study), patients with type 2 diabetes randomized to atorvastatin daily had an ~36% significant reduction in major cardiovascular events including stroke. In the Steno-2 study, a target-driven, intensified intervention aimed at multiple cardiovascular risk factors (glucose, lipids, and blood pressure), the risk of cardiovascular and microvascular events was reduced by ~50% and prompted long-term reductions in mortality.

Aspirin therapy

Low-dose aspirin was demonstrated to be effective in reducing MIs in subjects without diabetes in the Physician's Health Study and in multiple other studies. A meta-analysis of 145 controlled trials of antiplatelet therapy showed that both men and women had a significant reduction in vascular events. The Early Treatment Diabetic Retinopathy Study demonstrated the safety of aspirin therapy in people with diabetes and retinopathy and also found a reduction in MI risk. As a result of these findings, the American Diabetes Association recommends aspirin therapy for all people with diabetes who have evidence of macrovascular disease and consideration of aspirin therapy for individuals who are age >40 years and at high risk because of family history, smoking, hypertension, albuminuria, obesity, and/or dyslipidemia, unless there is a contraindication. Enteric-coated aspirin in doses of 75–162 mg daily is recommended. Adjunctive therapy with clopidogrel may be considered in high-risk subjects or aspirin-intolerant patients. Aspirin should not be used in individuals under age 21 years because of increased risk of Reye's syndrome.

Management of hypertension

There is incontrovertible evidence that hypertension complicating diabetes increases the risk of microvascular complications, cardiovascular events, and death. Epidemiologic analyses have demonstrated that blood pressure levels >115/75 mmHg are associated with increased cardiovascular events and mortality in diabetes. Control of hypertension in individuals with diabetes reduces the development and progression of coronary heart disease events, stroke, and nephropathy. Treatment of hypertension in diabetic patients should be vigorous.

Several major randomized clinical trials such as UKPDS, Hypertension Optimal Treatment (HOT), or Heart Outcomes Prevention Evaluation (HOPE) demonstrated that tight control of blood pressure was particularly beneficial in patients with diabetes in reducing major cardiovascular events.

The UKPDS explored the benefits of blood pressure lowering with captopril or atenolol on microvascular and macrovascular end points in subjects with type 2 diabetes and found that a 10/5 mmHg systolic/diastolic blood pressure reduction lowered the incidence of microvascular complications by 37%. Major cardiovascular events, including death, were reduced by 32%. In this study, the greatest benefits were observed in subjects achieving both glycemic *and* hypertension control. These results have been duplicated in more than a half-dozen studies using thiazide diuretics, angiotensin-converting enzyme (ACE) inhibitors, angiotensin receptor blockers (ARBs), β-blockers, and calcium-channel blockers (CCBs).

A recent meta-analysis of 27 randomized trials has suggested that different classes of blood pressure–lowering agents offer similar levels of reduction of cardiovascular risk. However, in diabetes, lower blood pressure goals appear to result in greater reductions of major cardiovascular events. It is therefore recommended that patients with diabetes should be treated to a systolic blood pressure <130 mmHg and diastolic blood pressure <80 mmHg, goals that should be implemented through a combined multidisciplinary approach.

Current recommendations are outlined in Table 5.2. Before initiating therapy, hypertension should be confirmed by repeat measurements. Automated ambulatory blood pressure monitoring may be especially helpful in people with diabetes, who often lose nocturnal blood pressure reduction. Autonomic dysfunction and orthostatic hypotension in individuals with longstanding diabetes or with symptoms should be excluded by measuring supine, sitting, and standing blood pressure. In individuals with mild hypertension (130–139/80–89 mmHg), a short trial of lifestyle modification may be tried, including weight reduction, increased exercise, smoking cessation, and reduced alcohol and sodium intake. Institute pharmacological therapy if these interventions fail.

Pharmacotherapy of hypertension. Based on recent trials, some general recommendations for the treatment of hypertension in people with diabetes have emerged. ACE inhibitors, ARBs, β-blockers, diuretics, and calcium-channel antagonists have all been shown to reduce cardiovascular events in diabetes. The selection of individual agents depends on the clinical characteristics of the individual, but there are cautions because of diabetes. In particular, elderly patients with diabetes should have their blood pressure lowered gradually, because they can experience significant hypotension on initiation of therapy. Commonly, two or more drugs are needed to adequately control hypertension in this population.

All subjects with diabetes requiring antihypertensive therapy should be treated with a regimen that includes an ACE inhibitor or an ARB. ACE inhibitors and ARBs are attractive choices because they have unique renal protective effects (of particular importance in people with diabetes) and, in some studies, have demonstrated a benefit of reducing CVD risk compared with other agents and/or independent

Table 5.2 Blood Pressure Targets in Individuals with Diabetes

	Systolic Blood Pressure	Diastolic Blood Pressure
Goal (mmHg)	<130	<80
Behavioral therapy alone (maximum 3 months), then add pharmacological treatment	130–139	80–89
Behavioral therapy + pharmacological treatment	≥140	≥90

of blood pressure–lowering effects. However, some caution is appropriate. Renal insufficiency may worsen in patients with bilateral renal artery stenosis, a problem that may be silent and more common in type 2 diabetes. Diabetic nephropathy is associated with hyporeninemic hypoaldosteronism, and ACE inhibitors and ARBs may cause unacceptable hyperkalemia in these patients. ARBs may be substituted for an ACE inhibitor if unacceptable side effects occur; these agents tend to cause less hyperkalemia and cough.

Based on multiple studies, a thiazide diuretic such as hydrochlorothiazide or chlorthalidone (25 mg/day) should be used among the first two drugs for managing hypertension in patients with diabetes. The benefit of thiazide diuretics may be particularly large in African-American patients. Rare patients will exhibit significant deterioration in glycemic control, particularly if hypokalemia complicates diuretic therapy. In patients with diabetes and refractory hypertension, more intensive diuresis using the addition of loop diuretics to reduce intravascular volume can be particularly effective, especially in patients with renal insufficiency or evidence of volume overload. Caution is necessary when initiating ACE inhibitor therapy in patients on diuretics because hypotension may occur.

Patients with diabetes and prior MI, angina, or congestive heart failure should be treated with a β-blocker, since these agents have been shown to reduce the risk of death. Treatment with some β-blockers can result in worsening of glycemic control, which can easily be overcome with modification of the diabetes treatment program. For this reason, β-blockers that block both β- and α1-adrenergic receptors and are metabolically neutral may be preferred. β-Blockers have also been suggested to reduce symptoms of hypoglycemia by interfering with adrenergic responses. Patients should be counseled in this regard, but β-blockers should not be withheld in patients with coronary disease or heart failure, except potentially in the setting of documented severe hypoglycemia.

CCBs are among the most effective blood pressure–lowering agents. As monotherapy in head-to-head studies, they have generally had more modest effects on CVD risk than the other classes listed above. However, verapamil and the dihydropyridine CCBs clearly have a place in combination with ACE inhibitors and ARBs in treating hypertension and reducing CVD risk in diabetes. Combination therapy of CCBs and ARBs can reduce the peripheral edema associated with CCB monotherapy.

Central sympatholytic agents may worsen orthostatic hypotension and sexual dysfunction. Peripheral α-blockers as monotherapy have been associated with a higher risk of congestive heart failure than thiazide diuretics and should not be used as first-line therapy in managing hypertension.

Direct renin inhibition is now possible using aliskirin, which unlike ACE inhibitors and ARBs, lowers plasma renin activity. This has been shown to be effective in lowering blood pressure in combination with the ACE inhibitor ramipril in type 2 diabetes.

Management of dyslipidemia

In type 2 diabetes, an increased prevalence of lipid abnormalities contributes to accelerated atherosclerosis. Characteristically, triglyceride-rich VLDL levels are elevated, and HDL cholesterol levels, particularly the larger, more beneficial

HDL2, are decreased. LDL cholesterol levels are usually not different from those found in age- and sex-matched individuals without diabetes, but the LDL particles may be smaller and denser, more oxidized, and glycated, all of which increase their atherogenicity. Associated obesity aggravates the lipid abnormalities. This lipid profile is the result of a combination of altered synthesis, catabolism, and clearance. A fasting lipid profile is recommended at initial evaluation and at least annually in adults with type 2 diabetes. In adults with low-risk lipid values (HDL cholesterol >60 mg/dl, triglycerides <150 mg/dl, and LDL cholesterol <100 mg/dl), repeat assessments can be performed every 2 years.

The Adult Treatment Panel (ATP) III subcommittee of the National Cholesterol Education Program (NCEP) recommendations for the screening and treatment of dyslipidemia are based predominantly on clinical studies in populations without diabetes. The American Diabetes Association has made some minor modifications to these recommendations specific for people with diabetes because of the high risk of atherosclerosis and the difference in the dyslipidemia commonly found.

- All patients with type 2 diabetes should be screened for dyslipidemia during their initial evaluation by measuring a fasting lipid profile, including triglycerides, total cholesterol, HDL cholesterol, and calculated LDL cholesterol. Triglyceride levels elevated >400 mg/dl, common in individuals with type 2 diabetes, invalidates the calculated LDL cholesterol level.
- The increased relative risk for CVD in both men and women with type 2 diabetes and the common coexisting risk factors (e.g., hypertension) place most adults with type 2 diabetes in a high-risk category.
- Lifestyle modification with reduction of saturated fat, *trans* fat, and cholesterol intake, weight loss, increased physical activity, and smoking cessation is very important, particularly in reducing triglycerides and increasing HDL cholesterol.
- Lowering LDL cholesterol to <100 mg/dl is the primary goal of therapy. For patients >40 years of age, statin therapy to achieve an LDL reduction of 30–40% regardless of baseline LDL levels is recommended.

Lipid level goals for adults with diabetes are given in Table 5.3. Recent clinical trials in high-risk patients, such as those with acute coronary syndromes or previous

Table 5.3 Lipoprotein Level Goals for Adults with Diabetes

	Lipids
LDL cholesterol*	<100 mg/dl (<2.6 mmol/l) <70 mg/dl (<3.9 mmol/l) optional in high-risk patients
HDL cholesterol	>40 mg/dl (>1.1 mmol/l) for men, >50 mg/dl (>1.3 mmol/l) for women are ideal
Triglycerides†	<150 mg/dl (<1.7 mmol/l) is ideal

*Current ADA guidelines recommend statin therapy to achieve an LDL reduction of 30–40%, regardless of baseline.
†Current NCEP/ATP III guidelines suggest that in patients with triglycerides ≥200 mg/dl, the "non-HDL cholesterol" (total cholesterol – HDL cholesterol) be used. The goal is ≤130 mg/dl.

cardiovascular events, have demonstrated that more aggressive therapy with high doses of statins to achieve an LDL of <70 mg/dl led to a significant reduction in further events. The risk of side effects with high doses of statins is outweighed by the benefits of such therapy in these high-risk patients. Therefore, a reduction in LDL to a goal of <70 mg/dl is an option in very-high-risk patients with overt CVD.

In many cases, elevated triglyceride levels can be satisfactorily lowered by improving glycemic control with nutrition therapy, exercise, oral agents, or insulin. Nutrition recommendations for these patients include a moderate increase in mono-unsaturated fat intake, with <10% of calories from saturated and polyunsaturated fats, and a more moderate intake of carbohydrate. A triglyceride level significantly >500 mg/dl is considered a risk factor for pancreatitis and should be aggressively managed. Such patients need to reduce intake of all types of dietary fat to lower levels of plasma dietary fat as chylomicrons, need aggressive glycemic control, and often need pharmacotherapy specifically targeting triglycerides (fibrate, niacin, or fish oil).

Pharmacotherapy of hyperlipidemia. When aggressive diet, exercise, and glucose control fail to control hyperlipidemia, the addition of LDL cholesterol–lowering drugs or triglyceride-lowering drugs, depending on the lipid profile, is indicated. Treatment of elevated LDL cholesterol is considered to have first priority, and LDL cholesterol should be lowered to <100 mg/dl. Subgroup analysis of the subjects with diabetes in large trials of the HMG CoA-reductase inhibitors (statins) such as the Heart Protection Study has shown these agents to be effective in reducing cardiovascular events independent of baseline LDL, preexisting vascular disease, type or duration of diabetes, or adequacy of glycemic control. Similarly, the CARDS patients with type 2 diabetes randomized to atorvastatin daily had a significant reduction in cardiovascular events including stroke.

Statins are also the most effective LDL cholesterol–lowering medications available and have an excellent safety profile. In high doses, some statins also reduce triglycerides significantly. Recent studies using statins suggest that lowering LDL cholesterol to 60–70 mg/dl further benefits people, including those with type 2 diabetes, with prior MI, compared with lowering LDL cholesterol to 96 mg/dl. Thus, it appears that aggressive lowering of LDL cholesterol levels with high-dose statin therapy may provide additional benefit to reduce heart disease in high-risk populations. In patients who do not achieve LDL cholesterol targets as a result of statin intolerance or for other reasons, bile-acid sequestrants and cholesterol absorption inhibitors can be used to further reduce LDL cholesterol levels. However, no evidence exists as to whether such combination therapy is more effective than a statin alone in preventing cardiovascular events.

Fibrates, particularly fenofibrate, and nicotinic acid can reduce LDL cholesterol levels as well but are primarily used to lower triglyceride and raise HDL cholesterol levels. Fibrates and nicotinic acid are associated with a low-level risk of rhabdomyolysis when combined with statins; this risk seems to be lower with fenofibrate than with gemfibrozil and higher at higher doses of statins. Nicotinic acid at moderate doses (750–2,000 mg/day) has been shown to only modestly increase glucose levels in the setting of diabetes; this can usually be managed by adjusting antihyperglycemic therapy.

Nicotinic acid and fibrates both increase HDL cholesterol and lower triglyceride levels and have been demonstrated to decrease cardiovascular morbidity in clinical trials that excluded or had very few patients with type 2 diabetes. In the VA-HIT study, gemfibrozil treatment was associated with a reduction in cardiovascular events in patients with diabetes, clinical CVD, and low HDL cholesterol and near-normal LDL cholesterol levels. In the Fenofibrate Intervention and Event Lowering in Diabetes (FIELD) study, fenofibrate reduced total cardiovascular events, nonfatal myocardial infarctions, and revascularizations but did not significantly affect mortality. Combination therapy using statins and fibrates or niacin may be necessary to achieve lipid targets, but have not been evaluated in outcomes studies for either event reduction or safety. Triglyceride levels significantly >500 mg/dl are considered a risk factor for pancreatitis and should be aggressively managed. In the presence of dyslipidemia characterized predominantly by severely elevated triglycerides, a fibrate is recommended, but additional therapy with nicotinic acid and omega-3 fatty acids (2–4 g/day) may be required.

Smoking cessation

Cigarette smoking is associated with accelerated macrovascular disease, and the presence of diabetes in a patient who smokes will further increase that individual's risk. Ongoing efforts should be made by the practitioner to assist the patient in discontinuing cigarette smoking, including enrollment in formal smoking cessation programs, behavioral modification, and use of nicotine patches. Some individuals may benefit from a trial of bupropion HCl or varenicline to relieve some withdrawal symptoms.

TREATMENT OF CARDIOVASCULAR DISEASE

Clinical trials that examined the efficacy of secondary interventions (after clinical disease has occurred) have often excluded patients with diabetes. However, clinical experience and a limited number of trials in type 2 diabetes suggest efficacy of medical and surgical treatments of cardiac, cerebral, and peripheral arterial disease similar to those in nondiabetic populations, with several caveats. Anti-anginal treatment regimens and treatment of other risk factors after an MI probably provide a similar benefit to both people with and without diabetes. Clinical trials such as the Norwegian timolol study have included a sufficient number of patients with type 2 diabetes to demonstrate efficacy of β-blockade in preventing a second MI. In insulin- or sulfonylurea-treated patients, the heightened risks of hypoglycemia with β-blockade must be taken into account.

Despite the generally more diffuse coronary and peripheral artery disease in patients with type 2 diabetes compared with patients without diabetes, bypass surgery is an effective treatment, although patients with diabetes do have increased morbidity and mortality. The Bypass Angioplasty Revascularization Investigation found that patients with multiple vessel disease had much better survival when randomized to coronary artery bypass grafting, including internal mammary artery grafting, than did patients undergoing angioplasty. It is not known whether the superiority of surgical approaches will also apply to patients with more focal disease or whether the use of newer stents and glycoprotein IIa/IIIb inhibitors during percutaneous intervention during angioplasty will minimize the differences in outcomes between the two approaches. Studies suggest that glycemic control before and during interventional coronary vessel procedures improves overall patient outcomes.

DIABETIC RETINOPATHY

The importance of frequent evaluation of and early detection and treatment of vision problems in patients with diabetes is illustrated by the following points:

- ~5,000 new cases of blindness related to diabetes are estimated to occur every year in the U.S., making diabetes the leading cause of new blindness among adults age 20–74 years.
- >60% of patients with type 2 diabetes have some degree of retinopathy 20 years after diagnosis. At the same point, nearly all patients with type 1 diabetes have retinopathy.
- Up to 21% of patients with type 2 diabetes have retinopathy at diagnosis.
- Loss of vision associated with proliferative retinopathy and macular edema can, if identified in a timely manner, be reduced by 50% with laser photocoagulation.
- Aspirin therapy does not prevent retinopathy or increase the risk of hemorrhage.

As in type 1 diabetes, the development and progression of retinopathy in type 2 diabetes is duration dependent and associated with higher glycemic levels. Keeping glycemia in the near-normal range definitely prevents or delays the onset of retinopathy. High blood pressure is a risk factor for the development of macular edema and is associated with the presence of proliferative retinopathy. Lowering blood pressure decreases the progression of retinopathy. Attempts to normalize glucose and blood pressure levels are appropriate. Although relatively fewer people with type 2 diabetes versus type 1 diabetes develop proliferative retinopathy, macular edema may be more common. In addition to retinopathy, patients with type 2 diabetes develop cataracts more frequently and at an earlier age than do people without diabetes.

Diabetic retinopathy does not cause visual symptoms until at a fairly advanced stage, usually when either proliferative retinopathy or macular edema is present. Management is more satisfactory when intervention is undertaken before visual symptoms develop. Therefore, yearly ophthalmoscopic examination by an ophthalmologist or optometrist who is experienced in diagnosing diabetic retinopathy is of crucial importance.

The frequency of visual impairment related to diabetes makes effective patient education crucial. Table 5.4 presents patient teaching points concerning retinopathy.

STAGES OF DIABETIC RETINOPATHY

Nonproliferative diabetic retinopathy

Nonproliferative diabetic retinopathy is the earliest stage and is characterized by microaneurysms and intraretinal "dot and blot" hemorrhages. Most individuals with long-term type 2 diabetes eventually develop it, but in many cases, it does not progress and has no effect on visual acuity. However, if the abnormal vessels leak serous fluid in the area of the maculae, which is responsible for central vision, macular edema

Table 5.4 What Patients Need to Know—Retinopathy

- Inform newly diagnosed patients that vision loss is a possibility and that they must report visual symptoms promptly.
- Instruct patients regarding the relationship between hyperglycemia, hypertension, and diabetic retinopathy, focusing on risk factor control to preserve eyesight.
- Ensure that patients understand the importance of an annual dilated eye examination by an ophthalmologist or optometrist because retinopathy outcomes are better with early detection and treatment.
- Reassure patients concerning transient vision changes associated with casual glycemic fluctuations and temporary changes in retinopathy status due to changes in glycemic therapy or pregnancy.
- Inform patients of the sight-saving procedures, including photocoagulation, available for severe nonproliferative and proliferative retinopathy and macular edema.
- Inform patients that isometric exercises that raise intra-ocular pressure can aggravate proliferative retinopathy.
- Suggest support programs and community services for patients with visual impairments or blindness.

can occur, with disruption of the usual transmission of light, and result in a decrease in visual acuity. Macular edema may be mild and not immediately threaten vision or may be clinically significant and require treatment because of the immediate threat to central vision. The presence of macular edema is suspected if there are hard exudates in close proximity to the maculae. Circinate hard exudates near the maculae are especially suspicious. Any of these findings should prompt referral to an ophthalmologist with expertise in treating diabetic retinopathy.

Severe nonproliferative retinopathy

Certain retinal lesions represent an advanced form of nonproliferative retinopathy. These lesions include cotton-wool spots (also referred to as soft exudates), which are ischemic infarcts in the inner retinal layers; "beading" of the retinal veins; and intraretinal microvascular abnormalities, which are dilated, tortuous retinal capillaries, or perhaps newly formed vessels within the retina. When these lesions are found together, the risk of progression to the proliferative stage is increased, and presence of any of these signs should prompt referral to an ophthalmologist who is knowledgeable and experienced in the management of diabetic retinopathy.

Proliferative diabetic retinopathy

The most vision-threatening stage of diabetic retinopathy is characterized by neovascularization on the surface of the retina, sometimes extending into the posterior vitreous. These vessels probably develop in response to ischemia. The prevalence of proliferative retinopathy among people who have had type 2 diabetes for >20 years may approach 30%. Proliferative retinopathy threatens vision because the new vessels are prone to bleed, especially if they are stretched by contraction of the vitreous. If bleeding into the preretinal space or vitreous occurs, the patient is likely to report "floaters" or "cobwebs" in the field of vision. The patient who has a major retinal hemorrhage will experience a sudden, painless loss of vision. The proliferation of fibrous tissue that often follows can lead to retinal detachment as fibrous tissue contracts.

PREVENTION OF VISION LOSS FROM RETINOPATHY

Both the Diabetes Control and Complications Trial (DCCT) and the UKPDS demonstrated that intensive treatment that lowers average glucose levels to near normal prevents or ameliorates retinopathy. Additionally, the small Kumamoto study in Japan demonstrated benefit of improved control in type 2 diabetic patients, and the Wisconsin Epidemiologic Study of Diabetic Retinopathy found a strong association between baseline glycated hemoglobin and progression of retinopathy in type 2 diabetic patients independent of treatment. Also, two large prospective studies, the Diabetic Retinopathy Study and the Early Treatment of Diabetic Retinopathy Study, provided strong support for the benefits of photocoagulation therapy, which decreases loss of vision in patients with proliferative retinopathy or macular edema. Therefore, timely identification of patients at risk is a major means of preventing vision loss.

The UKPDS also provided evidence that blood pressure control prevents the appearance and progression of retinopathy, although the Appropriate Blood Pressure Control in Diabetes Trial did not confirm a difference in retinopathy between intensive and moderate blood pressure control. Given the known benefits of blood pressure control on cardiovascular and other microvascular outcomes (such as nephropathy), good blood pressure control remains a prudent recommendation.

Evaluation and referral

Because the changes involved in diabetic retinopathy may be subtle and can escape detection by direct ophthalmoscopy, all patients with type 2 diabetes should have an annual examination with complete visual history, visual acuity examination, and careful dilated pupil ophthalmoscopic examination by an ophthalmologist or optometrist. The evaluations should begin at diabetes diagnosis, because the duration of hyperglycemia before diagnosis of type 2 diabetes is uncertain, and many patients already have retinopathy at diagnosis. The indications for referral are listed in Table 5.5. Note that 25–50% of patients with any high-risk characteristic may sustain severe visual loss within 2 years unless photocoagulation treatment is performed. Although nondilated photographic retinal screening is available, it is not a replacement for the annual examination because no rigorous studies have demonstrated equivalent diagnostic accuracy, and screening (such as for glaucoma) cannot be carried out.

Note that visual acuity changes are frequently related to fluctuating glycemic levels and corresponding changes in hydration of the crystalline lens. Thus, a presenting symptom of diabetes in a patient may be a change in vision. Likewise, a patient whose glycemic levels are decreased in response to proper treatment may experience visual acuity changes and should be forewarned as well as reassured that these will resolve over time.

Table 5.5 Indications for Referral of Patients with Type 2 Diabetes to Ophthalmologist or Optometrist

- High-risk patients—immediate referral to an ophthalmologist
  - Neovascularization covering more than one-third of optic disk
  - Vitreous or preretinal hemorrhage with any neovascularization, particularly on optic disk
  - Macular edema
- Symptomatic patients
  - Blurry vision persisting for >1–2 days not associated with change in blood glucose
  - Sudden loss of vision in one or both eyes
  - Black spots, cobwebs, or flashing lights in field of vision
- Asymptomatic patients
  - Annual examinations
  - Hard exudates near macula
  - Any preproliferative or proliferative characteristics
  - Pregnancy

TREATMENT OF RETINOPATHY

The ophthalmologic treatment of diabetic retinopathy depends on the stage of disease. There is no commonly accepted therapy for nonproliferative retinopathy other than improved glycemic and blood pressure control. Panretinal photocoagulation is considered the treatment of choice for patients who have proliferative retinopathy with high-risk characteristics, and it reduces the risk of severe visual loss by ~60%. Photocoagulation slows progressive visual loss in patients with macular edema by 50%.

Photocoagulation is used to stop neovascularization before recurrent hemorrhages into the vitreous cause irreparable damage. Sometimes photocoagulation is used to treat eyes with proliferative retinopathy before high-risk characteristics have developed. However, the risks of photocoagulation are such that usually only one eye is treated; treatment of the other eye is deferred unless high-risk characteristics develop. If retinal detachment and massive vitreous hemorrhage occur, closed vitrectomy can be used to remove bloody vitreous and bands of fibrous tissue. During the procedure, clear fluid is infused to replace vitreous, and traction on the retina is relieved. In ~50–65% of cases, some sight can be restored with this procedure.

DIABETIC RENAL DISEASE

Diabetic nephropathy occurs in 20–40% of individuals with diabetes and is the leading cause of ESRD. More than 40% of new cases of ESRD, >40,000 annually, are due to diabetes. The incidence of ESRD is four times higher in African Americans, four to six times higher in Mexican Americans, and six times higher in Native Americans than in whites with type 2 diabetes. The frequency of kidney disease related to diabetes makes effective patient education crucial. Table 5.6 presents patient teaching points concerning nephropathy.

CLINICAL PRESENTATION OF NEPHROPATHY

The development of diabetic nephropathy is asymptomatic, and its detection relies on laboratory screening. The usual course of diabetic nephropathy in type 2 diabetes is not as stereotypical as in type 1 diabetes, but nephropathy tends to progress through several defined stages. The first sign of developing nephropathy is the occurrence of elevated albumin excretion (>30 mg albumin/24 h or spot albumin/creatinine >30 mg/g). Whether microalbuminuria carries the same risk for the eventual development of clinical nephropathy in type 2 diabetes as seems to be the case in type 1 diabetes is unclear. As nephropathy progresses, "clinical" (dipstick positive, >300 mg albuminuria/24 h) proteinuria occurs. In contrast to type 1 diabetes, hypertension usually is present before the development of clinical proteinuria. In addition, a significant proportion of type 2 diabetic patients can develop renal insufficiency without significant albuminuria. Eventually, nephrotic-range proteinuria develops, followed by decreasing glomerular filtration rate (GFR) with rising serum creatinine, until ESRD occurs.

The importance of early identification is emphasized by evidence that intervention can lead to regression or remission of microalbuminuria, whereas overt proteinuria (urine microalbumin excretion >300 mg/day) is far more difficult to reverse. Nevertheless, specific interventions when overt proteinuria exists have been proven to reduce the incidence of kidney failure. Future approaches to early identification may include genetic screening for susceptibility loci and evaluation for early urinary biomarkers of diabetic renal disease.

CONDITIONS THAT INFLUENCE RENAL FUNCTION

Despite efforts at prevention, ~20–30% of all diabetic patients will develop some degree of nephropathy by 10 years after diagnosis. In patients with diabetes,

Table 5.6 What Patients Need to Know—Nephropathy

- Optimizing glycemic control prevents or delays nephropathy.
- Annual urine and blood tests are the only way to detect the "silent" onset of diabetic kidney disease.
- Regular blood pressure checks are vital because untreated hypertension damages the kidney, precipitates the onset of renal disease, and accelerates its progression.
- Effectively treating hypertension, with medication, weight loss, and/or sodium restriction, will help prevent or slow the progression of diabetic kidney disease.
- People with diabetes have an increased risk for urinary tract infections. Inform patients of the symptoms they need to detect and report.
- If there are signs of progressive nephropathy, explain the course of the disease and the options for treatment with dialysis and renal transplantation.

several conditions either precipitate the development of nephropathy or exacerbate the condition when present.

- **Hypertension** may precipitate the onset or further accelerate the process of renal insufficiency, or both. Virtually all patients with diabetes who develop nephropathy develop hypertension.
- **Neurogenic bladder** may predispose the patient to acute urinary retention or to moderate and persistent obstructive nephropathy. In either case, renal failure may be accelerated.
- When **infection and urinary obstruction** occur together, the risk of pyelonephritis and papillary necrosis increases, and this may result in a decline of renal function. Repetitive urethral instrumentation increases the risk of urinary tract infections. Infarction of the renal medulla and papillae can occur from ischemic necrosis and infarction or obstruction and is typically accompanied by fever, flank pain, anuria, and accelerated loss of renal function.
- **Nephrotoxic drugs,** such as nonsteroidal anti-inflammatory drugs, chronic analgesic abuse, and contrast media used in radiographic studies, have been associated with increased incidence and acceleration of renal failure in patients with diabetes. Nephrotoxic drugs should be avoided, and contrast media studies should be performed only after careful consideration of alternative procedures and with adequate hydration.

PREVENTION AND TREATMENT OF DIABETIC RENAL DISEASE

As with retinopathy, the DCCT and UKPDS demonstrated a decrease in development of microalbuminuria and clinical grade proteinuria with improved metabolic control. The UKPDS also showed that control of blood pressure reduces the risk for the development of nephropathy.

Three methods can be used for microalbuminuria screening: measurement of the albumin-to-creatinine ratio in a random spot collection; 24-h collection with creatinine, allowing the simultaneous measurement of creatinine clearance; or a timed (e.g., 4-h or overnight) collection. The spot measurement of the albumin-to-creatinine ratio is the easiest to perform and has a good predictive value. A value of >30 mg/g creatinine is considered abnormal. There is a diurnal variation, and the spot urine should be done in the morning if possible. A value for albumin excretion >30 mg/24 h is considered abnormal, as is a value >20 µg/min in a timed specimen. In addition to screening for microalbuminuria, a urinalysis (including microscopic analysis) and serum creatinine should be done in all newly diagnosed patients. Serum creatinine, with estimation of GFR, and urine albuminuria assessment should be repeated at least annually.

If present, infection should be treated before the significance of the proteinuria can be determined. The presence of microalbuminuria may be the first indication of advancing nephropathy and, if present, should prompt aggressive treatment of even modestly elevated blood pressure. To delay the onset and acceleration of renal disease in patients with diabetes, hypertension must be detected and treated aggressively. The ACE inhibitors and ARBs are particularly beneficial in this regard. In type 1 diabetes, ACE inhibitors have been shown to slow the progression of microalbuminuria to clinical proteinuria and the decline in GFR. In subjects with type 2 diabetes, ARBs have also been shown to reduce the risk of progression from micro-albuminuria to clinical proteinuria, as well as the latter to ESRD. ACE inhibitors and ARBs appear to provide equivalent efficacy, and recent literature suggests that combination use of an ACE inhibitor plus an ARB is safe and may provide synergistic renal benefits in diabetic patients. For this reason, guidelines advocate for the use of ACE inhibitors/ARBs, even in non-hypertensive patients with microalbuminuria. Dihydroperidine CCBs should only be used to achieve blood pressure targets in patients already treated with an ACE inhibitor or ARB. Although the Seventh Joint National Commission on High Blood Pressure (JNC 7), Kidney Disease Outcomes Quality Initiative (K/DOQI), and American Diabetes Association all recommend a target of <130/80 mmHg, analysis of some trials suggests that additional renal benefits may be achieved by lowering the systolic blood pressure to 120 mmHg.

There are potential complications associated with the use of antihypertensive medications to be kept in mind when instituting therapy.

Consultation with a specialist is suggested if there is progressive proteinuria or a decline in GFR, a GFR <60 ml/min, or hypertension unresponsive to multi-drug treatment. Nephrologists assist with patient education regarding renal disease, monitoring of renal disease progression, and blood pressure control. With further progression in renal insufficiency, the nephrologist's role expands to include managing the secondary complications such as anemia and secondary hyperparathyroidism, which typically develop in late stage 3 chronic kidney disease (estimated GFR <40 ml/min). In addition, the role of the dietitian becomes increasingly important in assisting with management of protein intake, hyperphosphatemia, hyperkalemia, and overall nutrition.

As diabetic patients approach end-stage renal failure, the nephrologist assumes a more central role in the coordination of care. The primary goals of management at this stage are transplantation evaluation and preparation for dialysis, usually in parallel. Early referral to a nephrologist (i.e., >3 months before initiation of dialysis) has been associated with higher vascular access rates, lower mortality on dialysis, and higher transplantation rates. Because preemptive renal transplantation occurs in <15% of cases, dialysis preparation remains imperative. This practice involves patient education and training, coordination of Medicare and insurance coverage, and choosing a dialysis center. Renal nurses and social workers play prominent roles in this process. Another key aspect of dialysis preparation is vascular access planning, which requires cooperation among nephrologists, radiologists, and surgeons to determine the best approach for each individual patient.

In summary, diabetic nephropathy is a complication with significant morbidity and mortality. Optimal management requires cooperation and coordination among several specialties, with the roles of each specialty evolving as disease progression occurs.

DIABETIC FOOT PROBLEMS

More than 50% of the nontraumatic amputations in the U.S. occur in individuals with diabetes, and it has been estimated that >50% of these amputations could have been prevented with proper care. Therefore, the clinician and patient who are conscientious about prevention, early detection, and prompt treatment of diabetic foot problems can make a significant impact on this complication.

CAUSES OF DIABETIC FOOT PROBLEMS

Foot lesions in individuals with diabetes are the result of polyneuropathy, peripheral arterial disease, superimposed infection, or, most often, a combination of these complications. Usually, lesions begin in feet that are insensitive, deformed, and/or ischemic. Such feet are susceptible to trauma, which may lead to callus formation, ulceration, infection, and gangrene.

In most patients with diabetes who have foot lesions, the primary pathophysiological event is the development of an insensitive foot secondary to polyneuropathy. Loss of foot sensation is often, but not always, accompanied by decreased vibratory sense and loss of ankle deep tendon reflexes. In addition to insensitivity, neuropathy may ultimately lead to a deformed foot secondary to tendon shortening (contractures), which leads to decreased mobility of the toes, abnormality in weight bearing, calluses, and development of classic "hammer toe" deformities. The combination of foot insensitivity and foot deformities that shift weight distribution promotes the development of foot ulcers. Neuropathy also causes decreased sweating and dry skin. If left untreated, cracked and thickened skin can lead to infections and ulcerations. Neuropathic ulcers in the patient with diabetes often go undetected because they are usually painless. Diabetic neuropathy is also associated with an increased risk of foot fractures, which is possibly increased by the use of thiazolidinediones.

Neuroarthropathy (Charcot arthropathy) is an underrecognized complication of diabetic neuropathy that can result in disabling foot deformities. It usually occurs in the presence of adequate circulation. It is characterized by disintegration and disorganization of the bones in the lower leg and foot and can be precipitated by minimal trauma. Early recognition and appropriate treatment (offloading and possibly bisphosphonates) can substantially reduce permanent deformities.

The sudden development of a painful distal foot lesion, usually secondary to trauma, may signify underlying peripheral arterial disease, which is associated with findings of decreased or absent pulses, dependent rubor, and pallor on elevation. The extent of the vascular disease and its potential for treatment by surgical intervention can be determined by Doppler noninvasive techniques and arteriography. Revascularization procedures, such as angioplasty and bypass, are often helpful in treating patients with severe, disabling claudication (at rest) or nonhealing ulcers or to aid healing of an amputation incision. Unfortunately, surgical intervention is not always effective in individuals with diabetes because many have diffuse vascular disease.

Infection is a frequent complication of both vascular and neuropathic ulcers. Studies indicate that these infections are often mixed and that gram-positive organisms predominate.

PREVENTION OF FOOT PROBLEMS

The prevention of foot problems in a person with diabetes requires proper foot care by the patient as well as early detection and prompt treatment of lesions by the physician. Help from other health care specialists (e.g., podiatrist, orthopedist, vascular surgeon, or experts in shoe fitting) is frequently needed.

The first step in prevention is to educate all patients and to identify those who need specialized or frequent evaluations because of risk factors for foot problems (Table 5.7). During the evaluation, the examiner should determine whether the

Table 5.7 What Patients Need to Know—Foot Care

- The patient, or family member in the case of a patient who is impaired by morbid obesity or blindness, has the major responsibility for prevention of foot problems.
- Cut toenails straight across and inspect the feet daily for cuts, abrasions, blisters, and corns.
- Regular washing with warm water and mild soap followed by thorough drying is essential.
- Use moistening agents, such as lanolin, as needed.
- Avoid prolonged soaking, strong chemicals such as Epsom salts or iodine, and "home surgery."
- Heat, cold, new shoes, constricting or mended socks, and, perhaps most important, going barefoot are potential hazards that must be emphasized to all patients, especially those with peripheral neuropathy.

patient has experienced foot problems or intermittent claudication since the last visit. The physician also should conduct a thorough examination of both feet, looking for the signs and symptoms of impending foot problems (Table 5.8), including foot deformities, calluses, and ulcers. The clinician should also check the pulses (dorsalis pedis, posterior, tibial, and femoral), search for bruits, and determine reflexes and sensation in the toes and feet. Evaluation of neurological status in the foot should involve the use of the Semmes-Weinstein 5.07 (10-g) monofilament (Table 5.9; Fig. 5.1) and 128-Hz tuning fork.

Table 5.8 Physician-Performed Monofilament Examination

- Examination must be done in a quiet and relaxed supine position.
- Have patients close their eyes.
- First, apply the monofilament on the patient's hands to teach him or her what to feel. The patient must not be able to see whether the filament is being applied.
- Three sites are tested on each foot: the big toe pulp and the first and fifth metatarsus heads.
- Apply the filament perpendicular to test the skin surface with sufficient force to cause the filament to bend ~45°; the entire procedure should take ~2 seconds.
- Ask patients *if* and *where* they felt pressure applied.
- Repeat the measurement twice at the each site per foot in random order.
- Express the result separately for each foot in a ratio, e.g., 4/6 means the patient felt 4 touches of 6; 6/6 means the patient felt each application.
- During the procedure, test twice by a blind application the patient's drive to comply with you. If the patient answers positively while no filament is applied, cancel everything, further explain this procedure and its importance, and repeat entire procedure.

Table 5.9 Warning Symptoms and Signs of Diabetic Foot Problems

	Symptoms	Signs
Vascular	Cold feet Intermittent claudication involving calf or foot Pain at rest, especially nocturnal, relieved by dependency	Absent pedal, popliteal, or femoral pulses Femoral bruits Dependent rubor, plantar pallor on elevation Prolonged capillary filling time (>3–4 seconds) Decreased skin temperature
Neurologic	*Sensory:* burning, tingling, or crawling sensations; pain and hypersensitivity, cold feet Hand symptoms *Motor:* weakness (foot drop) *Autonomic:* diminished sweating	*Sensory:* deficits (vibratory, light touch and proprioceptive, pain and temperature perception), hyperesthesia Carpal tunnel syndrome (paresthesiae, sensory loss over median distribution) *Motor:* diminished to absent deep tendon reflexes (Achilles, then patellar), weakness, wasting *Autonomic:* diminished to absent sweating Heat and edema due to increased arteriovenous shunting
Musculoskeletal	Gradual change in foot shape, sudden painless change in foot shape, with swelling, without history or trauma Weakness of hand muscles	Cavus feet with claw toes Drop foot "Rocker-bottom" foot Neuropathic arthropathy (Charcot's joint) Wasting
Dermatologic	Exquisitely painful or painless wounds Slow-healing or nonhealing wounds or necrosis Skin color changes (cyanosis, redness) Chronic scaling, itching or dry feet Recurrent infections (e.g., paronychia, athlete's foot)	*Skin:* Abnormal dryness Chronic tinea infections Keratotic lesions with or without hemorrhage (plantar or digital) Trophic ulcer *Hair:* Diminished or absent *Nails:* Trophic changes Onychomycosis Sublingual ulceration or abscess Ingrown nails with paronychia

TREATMENT OF FOOT PROBLEMS

Minor noninfected wounds can be treated with nonirritating antiseptic solution, daily dressing changes, and foot rest. More serious problems, such as foot deformities, infected lesions, and osteomyelitis, are best handled in consultation with specialists in diabetic foot care. Infected foot ulcers usually require intra-

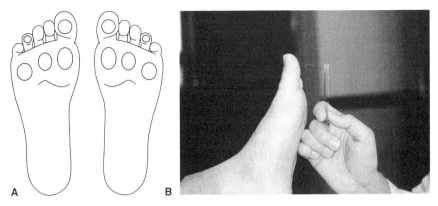

Figure 5.1 Sites (*A*) for Semmes-Weinstein monofilament testing (*B*).

venous antibiotics, bed rest with foot elevation, and surgical debridement. Reducing plantar pressure using contact casts/specialized footwear accelerates healing.

DIABETIC NEUROPATHIES

The diabetic neuropathies are among the most common and perplexing complications of diabetes. Neuropathy has a wide variety of manifestations in people with diabetes, and the descriptive terminology and classification have also varied, causing some confusion among clinicians. An accepted classification is presented in Table 5.10.

Table 5.10 Classification of Diabetic Neuropathies

- Distal symmetric sensorimotor polyneuropathy (DN)
- Autonomic neuropathy
- Focal and multifocal neuropathies
  - Cranial neuropathy
  - Limb mononeuropathy
    - Median
    - Ulnar
    - Radial
    - Femoral
    - Peroneal
    - Lateral femoral cutaneous
  - Trunk mononeuropathy
  - Mononeuropathy multiplex
  - Asymmetric lower-limb motor neuropathy (amyotrophy)
- Mixed forms

A complete dissertation on neuropathy is beyond the scope of this book section. Instead, a few important points about diagnosis and treatment of commonly encountered neuropathic problems are discussed.

Early recognition and appropriate management of neuropathy in patients with diabetes is important for a number of reasons: *1*) nondiabetic neuropathies may be present in patients with diabetes and may be treatable; *2*) a number of treatment options exist for symptomatic diabetic neuropathy; *3*) up to 50% of diabetic neuropathies may be asymptomatic, and patients are at risk of insensate injury to their feet; *4*) autonomic neuropathy may involve every system in the body; and *5*) cardiovascular autonomic neuropathy causes substantial morbidity and mortality.

Diabetic neuropathy begins as a generalized asymptomatic dysfunction of sensorimotor or autonomic peripheral nerve fibers and is by far the most common form. The sensorimotor neuropathy is symmetric and first involves the distal lower extremities. Symptoms vary according to the class of sensory fibers involved. The most common symptoms are tingling and pain which are induced by the involvement of small fibers. The pain is particularly troubling to most patients and is often the reason why patients with neuropathy seek medical care. Loss of feeling may also occur in the feet with or without pain or dysesthesias. If nociceptive fibers are involved, loss of sensation may set the stage for painless injuries.

The presence and severity of the neuropathy generally relates to the duration of diabetes and degree of hyperglycemia. In people with type 2 diabetes, neuropathy may be present at diagnosis. Painful neuropathy has been also identified in subjects with impaired glucose tolerance. Diabetic neuropathy is often associated with retinopathy and nephropathy. Both symptoms and deficits may have an adverse effect on quality of life in patients with neuropathy.

DIAGNOSIS AND TREATMENT OF NEUROPATHY

Several stages in the progression of neuropathy have been identified. The first abnormality might comprise an asymptomatic change in nerve conduction or reduction of the heartbeat response to deep breathing or the Valsalva maneuver. To define neuropathy, the changes should be present in two or more nerves. Next, the patient is found to have decreased or absent ankle reflexes and/or abnormal vibratory sensation of the great toes. When present, symptoms can be either pain or a loss of function. The pain intensity varies from causing discomfort to being disabling and may be described as sticking, lacinating, prickling, burning, aching, boring, and/or excessively sensitive. Fortunately, most patients do not have pain, and when present, the pain may be a transitory phase.

All patients should be screened for diabetic neuropathy at diagnosis and at least annually thereafter, using simple clinical tests. The Michigan Neuropathy Screening Instrument (MNSI) and similar symptom scoring systems are useful in clinical practice. Quantitative sensory testing is an additional measure to assess the loss of protective sensation (i.e., perceptions of light touch or pressure, vibration, heat and cold, and pain) and axonal pathology. Electrophysiological testing and specialized neurology evaluation may be needed in situations where the clinical features are atypical. Screening for autonomic neuropathy can also be performed, although special electrophysiological testing for autonomic neuropathy is rarely needed. Once the diagnosis of diabetic neuropathy is established, special foot care is appropriate for insensate feet to decrease the risk of ulcers and amputation as discussed above.

Loss of pain does not necessarily imply improvement in the neuropathy. Functional loss is more common and is manifested by decreased tactile sense, lack of temperature discrimination, sensory loss, and muscle weakness. Inability to walk on the heels is a sign of more severe neuropathy. The muscular weakness may lead to foot deformity, such as hammertoes and abnormal weight-bearing. The insensitivity leads to neglect of injury and contributes to foot ulcers (neurotrophic ulcers) and Charcot's joint. Although polyneuropathy can affect the hands, most often, hand symptoms are caused by carpal tunnel syndrome or ulnar neuropathy.

Control of hyperglycemia represents the main goal in the prevention and management of neuropathy and should be implemented as discussed above. Epidemiologic observations have also suggested that other metabolic and vascular factors, including hypertension, contribute to the disease state, and intensive management of hypertension represents an additional goal.

AUTONOMIC NEUROPATHY

Diminished autonomic nerve function can cause a variety of symptoms. Autonomic polyneuropathy, which usually occurs in concert with peripheral sensorimotor neuropathy, includes gastroparesis, diabetic diarrhea, constipation, neurogenic bladder, gustatory sweating, impaired cardiovascular reflexes and orthostatic hypotension, sexual dysfunction in men, and dyspareunia in women. Clinically, autonomic neuropathy tends to appear late in the course of diabetes.

Gastroparesis

Severe symptomatic gastroparesis is uncommon in people with type 2 diabetes. The patient with gastroparesis may experience early satiety, nausea, vomiting, abdominal discomfort, and fluctuations of postprandial blood glucose levels secondary to delayed emptying or retention of gastric contents. Other upper gastrointestinal abnormalities must be excluded before making a diagnosis of gastroparesis. Gastric emptying studies may be necessary to confirm the diagnosis, but may not correlate with symptoms. However, significant hyperglycemia can temporarily delay gastric emptying, so glycemic control during the test should be monitored. Metoclopramide is often helpful in treating gastroparesis but may be associated with dyskinetic side effects. Erythromycin and nortryptyline have been shown to improve gastric emptying and benefit some patients. Domperidone is an investigational drug (available in Canada) that has been shown to be effective. Botulinum toxin injection through transient paralysis of the pylorus was reported to accelerate gastric emptying and improve symptoms of nausea and vomiting in small clinical trials. The role of gastric pacing remains unclear and controversial.

Diabetic diarrhea

Frequent passage of loose stools, particularly after meals and at night, marks the acute phase of this condition. Diabetic diarrhea tends to be intermittent and may alternate with constipation. Diphenoxylate, loperamide, and clonidine have been shown to be effective to some degree. Some patients respond to treatment with a broad-spectrum antibiotic such as tetracycline. In resistant cases, parenteral octreotide can be helpful.

Neurogenic bladder

Neurogenic bladder is characterized by a pattern of frequent, small voidings and incontinence and may progress to urinary retention. The demonstration of cystometric abnormalities and large residual urine volume are necessary for diagnosis. The patient with significant urinary retention may need to perform intermittent self-catheterization. Rarely, surgical intervention may be required if the patient does not respond to conservative medical measures, because chronic urinary retention may lead to infection.

Cardiovascular autonomic neuropathy

Cardiovascular autonomic neuropathy (CAN) may present as an increased resting heart rate, and there may be inadequate capacity to increase heart rate in response to physiological demands. CAN is associated with increased mortality in patients with diabetes.

Orthostatic hypotension

Patients with orthostatic hypotension may find relief by non-pharmacological treatments such as: *1*) avoidance of sudden changes in body posture to the head-up position; *2*) avoiding medications that aggravate hypotension, such as tricyclic antidepressants and phenothiazines; *3*) eating small, frequent meals to avoid the postprandial hypotension that may occur after a large carbohydrate-containing meal; *4*) avoiding activities that involve straining; *5*) elevation of the head of the bed; and *6*) wearing compression stockings.

There are several pharmacological agents that can be used for treating orthostatic hypotension. If fludrocortisone is prescribed, the initial dose should be 0.1 mg/day, and increases up to 0.4 mg/day should be made gradually. The drug should be used with particular caution in patients with cardiac disease or concomitant supine hypertension, because it causes sodium and water retention. Clonidine, a central $\alpha2$-receptor–blocking agent, has also been used to treat this condition. Midodine is a newer agent that has been shown to benefit some patients. Erythropoietin may improve standing blood pressure in patients with orthostatic hypotension. Caffeine may also improve orthostatic hypotension and attenuate postprandial hypotension in patients with autonomic failure.

Sexual dysfunction in men

Sexual dysfunction is a frequent occurrence in men with diabetes and usually manifests as lack of a firm, sustained erection. In most cases, libido and ejaculatory function are not affected, although retrograde ejaculation may be another feature of autonomic neuropathy. The measurement of nocturnal penile tumescence is sometimes used to determine whether the patient's erections during sleep are normal, borderline, or abnormally diminished for age. When psychological and endocrine causes of impotence have been ruled out, the use of 5′ phosphodiesterase inhibitors (i.e., sildanafil, vardenafil, tadalafil), vacuum devices, intrapenile injections of vasodilating substances (e.g., papaverine, phentolamine, prostaglandin), or intra-urethral insertion of medication (alprostadil) may allow the patient to resume sexual intercourse. The implantation of an inflatable or semirigid prosthesis is another option.

OTHER VARIETIES OF DIABETIC NEUROPATHY

In addition to symmetric polyneuropathy, people with diabetes are subject to a variety of other neuropathic syndromes. These syndromes include lumbosacral plexus neuropathies (also called femoral neuropathy or diabetic amyotrophy), truncal radiculopathy, upper-limb mononeuropathies (the entrapment neuropathies—carpal tunnel syndrome and ulnar neuropathy, which are more common in people with diabetes), and cranial neuropathy. These varieties of neuropathy are asymmetric and abrupt or subacute in onset and tend to follow a monophasic course with improvement over time. They may be more common in type 2 diabetes, and their association with hyperglycemia is less clear-cut than that of polyneuropathy. In some cases, there is evidence that ischemia or inflammation is involved. Patients often have more than one type of diabetic neuropathy.

Lumbosacral plexus neuropathy may present with abrupt onset of asymmetric lower-limb proximal muscle pain and weakness or, in its most severe form, with severe pain, wasting of the proximal muscles, and modest sensory involvement (diabetic amyotrophy). It is more common in men with type 2 diabetes. Prominent features include quadriceps involvement, atrophy of thigh muscles, and absent patellar tendon reflexes. Recovery usually occurs in several months to a year. However, the condition may recur contralaterally.

Extra-ocular muscle motor paralysis, particularly that innervated by the third and sixth cranial nerves, is the most noticeable of the cranial mononeuropathies. Patients can also develop peroneal (foot drop) and median or ulnar palsies. Spontaneous recovery in about 3–6 months is usual.

The diagnosis of a diabetic neuropathy is often easily made on clinical evaluation with little testing necessary. People with diabetes can have neuropathy unrelated to their diabetes. When the clinical features are not typical (i.e., unilateral, predominantly upper limb, rapidly progressive, mainly motor) or consistent with the duration of diabetes and presence of other complications, other causes of neuropathy should be excluded.

A major goal in neuropathy management is controlling pain if present. A large number of agents have been studied in both uncontrolled and controlled clinical trials. Treatment with tricyclic antidepressant medications such as nortryptyline, the selective dual serotonin/norepinephrine reuptake inhibitor duloxetine, or anti-seizure medications such as gabapentin, pregabalin, lamictal, or carbamezepine may be helpful in some patients with painful neuropathy. Duloxetine and pregabalin are the only agents listed with a U.S. Food and Drug Administration indication for diabetic neuropathy. Other successful treatments include tramadol and lidoderm patches. A topical cream, capsaicin, is variably effective. Aspirin, propoxyphene, and other analgesics should be prescribed as necessary for pain.

Narcotics have reduced efficacy and in general should be withheld until all other treatment modalities have been exhausted. In general, low-dose combination of two or more drugs is more effective than a single agent for better symptomatic relief with fewer adverse effects. Physical therapy methods of treatment are often helpful. Referral to a pain clinic may be necessary.

BIBLIOGRAPHY

Adler AI, Stevens RJ, Manley SE, Bilous RW, Cull CA, Holman RR: Development and progression of nephropathy in type 2 diabetes: the United Kingdom Prospective Diabetes Study (UKPDS 64). *Kidney Int* 63:225–232, 2003

Adler AI, Stratton IM, Neil HA, Yudkin JS, Mathews DR, Cull CA, Wright AD, Turner RC, Holman RR: Association of systolic blood pressure with macrovascular and microvascular complications of type 2 diabetes (UKPDS 36): prospective observational study. *BMJ* 321:412–419, 2000

American Diabetes Association: Aspirin therapy in diabetes (Position Statement). *Diabetes Care* 27 (Suppl. 1):S72–S73, 2004

Bax JJ, Young LH, Frye RL, Bonow RO, Steinberg HO, Barrett EJ: Screening for coronary artery disease in patients with diabetes. *Diabetes Care* 30:2729–2736, 2007

American Diabetes Association: Preventive foot care in diabetes (Position Statement). *Diabetes Care* 27 (Suppl. 1):S63–S64, 2004

American Diabetes Association: Standards of medical care in diabetes—2008. *Diabetes Care* 31 (Suppl. 1):S12–S54, 2008

Arauz-Pacheco C, Parrott MA, Raskin P: The treatment of hypertension in adult patients with diabetes mellitus (Technical Review). *Diabetes Care* 25:134–147, 2002

Astor BC, Eustace JA, Powe NR, Klag MJ, Sadler JH, Fink NE, Coresh J: Timing of nephrologist referral and arteriovenous access use: the CHOICE Study. *Am J Kidney Dis* 38:494–501, 2001

Bakris GL, Williams M, Dworkin L, Elliot WJ, Epstein M, Toto R, Tuttle K, Douglas J, Hsueh W, Sowers J: Preserving renal function in adults with hypertension and diabetes: a consensus approach. *Am J Kid Dis* 36:646–661, 2000

The BARI Investigators: Influence of diabetes on 5-year mortality and morbidity in a randomized trial comparing CABG and PTCA in patients with multivessel disease. *Circulation* 96:1761–1769, 1997

Barnett AH, Bain SC, Bouter P, Karlberg B, Madsbad S, Jervell J, Mustonen J: Angiotensin-receptor blockade versus converting-enzyme inhibition in type 2 diabetes and nephropathy. *N Engl J Med* 351:1952–1961, 2004

Boulton AJ, Vinik AI, Arezzo JC, Bril V, Feldman EL, Freeman R, Malik RA, Maser RE, Sosenko JM, Ziegler D: Diabetic neuropathies: a statement by the American Diabetes Association. *Diabetes Care* 28:956–962, 2005

Brenner BM, Cooper ME, de Zeeuw D, Keane WF, Mitch WE, Parving HH, Remuzzi G, Snapinn SM, Zhang Z, Shahinfar S: Effects of losartan on renal and cardiovascular outcomes in patients with nephropathy due to type 2 diabetes. *N Engl J Med* 345:861–869, 2001

Breyer JA: Diabetic nephropathy in insulin-dependent patients. *Am J Kidney Dis* 20:533–547, 1992

Cabezas-Cerrato J: The prevalence of clinical diabetic polyneuropathy in Spain: a study in primary care and hospital clinic groups: Neuropathy Spanish Study Group of the Spanish Diabetes Society (SDS). *Diabetologia* 41:1263–1269, 1998

Cannon CP, Braunwald E, McCabe CH, Rader DJ, Rouleau JL, Belder R, Joyal SV, Hill KA, Pfeffer MA, Skene AM: Intensive versus moderate lipid lowering with statins after acute coronary syndromes. *N Engl J Med* 350:1495–1504, 2004

Cass A, Cunningham J, Snelling P, Ayanian JZ: Late referral to a nephrologist reduces access to renal transplantation. *Am J Kidney Dis* 42:1043–1049, 2003

Chobanian AV, Bakris GL, Black HR, Cushman WC, Green LA, Izzo JL Jr, Jones DW, Materson BJ, Oparil S, Wright JT Jr, Roccella EJ, the National Heart, Lung, and Blood Institute Joint National Committee on Prevention, Detection, Evaluation, and Treatment of High Blood Pressure, the National High Blood Pressure Education Program Coordinating Committee: The Seventh Report of the Joint National Committee on Prevention, Detection, Evaluation, and Treatment of High Blood Pressure: the JNC 7 report. *JAMA* 289:2560–2572, 2003

DCCT/EDIC Research Group: Retinopathy and nephropathy in patients with type 1 diabetes four years after a trial of intensive therapy. *N Engl J Med* 342:381–389, 2000

DCCT Research Group: The effect of intensive treatment of diabetes on the development and progression of long-term complications in insulin-dependent diabetes mellitus. *N Engl J Med* 329:977–986, 1993

DCCT Research Group: The effect of intensive diabetes therapy on the development and progression of neuropathy. *Ann Intern Med* 122:561–568, 1995

Feldman EL, Stevens MJ, Russell JW, Greene DA: Somatosensory neuropathy. In *Ellenberg and Rifkin's Diabetes Mellitus.* Porte D Jr, Sherwin RS, Baron A, Eds. New York, NY, McGraw Hill, 2002, p. 771–788

Freeman R: Autonomic peripheral neuropathy. *Lancet* 365:1259–1270, 2005

Hansson L, Zanchetti A, Carruthers SG, Dahlof B, Elmfield D, Julius S, Manard J, Rahn KH, Wedel H, Westerling S: Effects of intensive blood-pressure lowering and low-dose aspirin on patients with hypertension: principal results of the Hypertension Optimal Treatment (HOT) randomized trial: HOT Study Group. *Lancet* 351:1755–1762, 1998

Heart Outcomes Prevention Evaluation (HOPE) Study Investigators: Effects of ramipril on cardiovascular outcomes in people with diabetes mellitus: results of the HOPE study and MICRO-HOPE study. *Lancet* 355:253–259, 2000

Heart Protection Study Collaborative Group: MRC/BHF Heart Protection Study of cholesterol-lowering with simvastatin in 5963 people with diabetes: a randomized placebo-controlled trial. *Lancet* 361:2005–2016, 2003

Jacobsen P, Andersen S, Jensen BR, Parving HH: Additive effect of ACE inhibition and angiotensin II receptor blockade in type I diabetic patients with diabetic nephropathy. *J Am Soc Nephrol* 14:992–999, 2003

Kasiske BL, Snyder JJ, Matas AJ, Ellison MD, Gill JS, Kausz AT: Preemptive kidney transplantation: the advantage and the advantaged. *J Am Soc Nephrol* 13:1358–1364, 2002

KDOQI Clinical Practice Guidelines and Clinical Practice Recommendations for Diabetes and Chronic Kidney Disease. *Am J Kidney Dis* 49:S12–S154, 2007

Khush KK, Waters DD, Bittner V, Deedwania PC, Kastelein JJ, Lewis SJ, Wenger NK: Effect of high-dose atorvastatin on hospitalizations for heart failure: subgroup analysis of the Treating to New Targets (TNT) study. *Circulation* 115:576–583, 2007

Laverman GD, Remuzzi G, Ruggenenti P: ACE inhibition versus angiotensin receptor blockade: which is better for renal and cardiovascular protection? *J Am Soc Nephrol* 15 (Suppl. 1):S64–S70, 2004

Lewis EJ, Hunsicker LG, Clarke WR, Berl T, Pohl MA, Lewis JB, Ritz E, Atkins RC, Rohde R, Raz I: Renoprotective effect of the angiotensin-receptor antagonist irbesartan in patients with nephropathy due to type 2 diabetes. *N Engl J Med* 345:851–860, 2001

Mueller PW, Rogus JJ, Cleary PA, Zhao Y, Smiles AM, Steffes MW, Bucksa J, Gibson TB, Cordovado SK, Krolewski AS, Nierras CR, Warram JH: Genetics of Kidneys in Diabetes (GoKinD) study: a genetics collection available for identifying genetic susceptibility factors for diabetic nephropathy in type 1 diabetes. *J Am Soc Nephrol* 17:1782–1790, 2006

National Cholesterol Education Program (NCEP) Expert Panel of Detection, Evaluation and Treatment of High Blood Cholesterol in Adults (Adult Treatment Panel III): Executive summary of the Third Report of the National Cholesterol Education Program (NCEP) Expert Panel on the Detection, Evaluation and Treatment of High Blood Cholesterol in Adults (Adult Treatment Panel III). *JAMA* 285:2486–2497, 2001

Nissen SE, Tuzcu EM, Schoenhagen P, Brown BG, Ganz P, Vogel RA, Crowe T, Howard G, Cooper CJ, Brodie B, Grines CL, DeMaria AN: Effect of intensive compared with moderate lipid-lowering therapy on progression of coronary atherosclerosis: a randomized controlled trial. *JAMA* 291:1071–1080, 2004

O'Brien IA, McFadden JP, Corrall RJ: The influence of autonomic neuropathy on mortality in insulin-dependent diabetes. *Q J Med* 79:495–502, 1991

Ohkubo Y, Kishikawa H, Araki E, Isami S, Motoyoshi S, Kojima Y, Furuyoshi N, Shichiri M: Intensive insulin therapy prevents the progression of diabetic microvascular complications in Japanese patients with non-insulin-dependent diabetes mellitus: a randomized prospective 6-year study. *Diabetes Res Clin Pract* 28:103–117, 1995

Perkins BA, Ficociello LH, Silva KH, Finkelstein DM, Warram JH, Krolewski AS: Regression of microalbuminuria in type 1 diabetes. *N Engl J Med* 348:2285–2293, 2003

Rao PV, Lu X, Standley M, Pattee P, Neelima G, Girisesh G, Dakshinamurthy KV, Roberts CT Jr, Nagalla SR: Proteomic identification of urinary biomarkers of diabetic nephropathy. *Diabetes Care* 30:629–637, 2007

Rathmann W, Ziegler D, Jahnke M, Haastert B, Gries FA: Mortality in diabetic patients with cardiovascular autonomic neuropathy. *Diabet Med* 10:820–824, 1993

Shepherd J, Barter P, Carmena R, Deedwania P, Fruchart JC, Haffner S, Hsia J, Breazna A, LaRosa J, Grundy S, Waters D: Effect of lowering LDL cholesterol substantially below currently recommended levels in patients with coronary heart disease and diabetes: the Treating to New Targets (TNT) study. *Diabetes Care* 29:1220–1226, 2006

Siao P, Cros DP: Quantitative sensory testing. *Phys Med Rehabil Clin N Am* 14:261–286, 2003

Tesfaye S, Chaturvedi N, Eaton SE, Ward JD, Manes C, Ionescu-Tirgoviste C, Witte DR, Fuller JH: Vascular risk factors and diabetic neuropathy. *N Engl J Med* 352:341–350, 2005

U.K. Prospective Diabetes Study (UKPDS) Group: Effect of intensive blood-glucose control with metformin on complications in overweight patients with type 2 diabetes (UKPDS 34). *Lancet* 352:854–865, 1998

U.K. Prospective Diabetes Study (UKPDS) Group: Intensive blood-glucose control with sulphonylureas or insulin compared with conventional treatment and risk of complications in patients with type 2 diabetes (UKPDS 33). *Lancet* 352:837–853, 1998

U.K. Prospective Diabetes Study Group: Tight blood pressure control and risk of macrovascular and microvascular complications of type 2 diabetes: UKPDS 38. *BMJ* 317:703–713, 1998

Vileikyte L: Psychological aspects of diabetic peripheral neuropathy. *Diabetes Review* 7:387–394, 1999

Winkelmayer WC, Owen WF Jr, Levin R, Avorn J: A propensity analysis of late versus early nephrologist referral and mortality on dialysis. *J Am Soc Nephrol* 14:486–492, 2003

Young MJ, Adams JE, Anderson GF, Boulton AJ, Cavanagh PR: Medial arterial calcification in the feet of diabetic patients and matched non-diabetic control subjects. *Diabetologia* 36:615–621, 1993

Behavior Change Strategies

Highlights
Behavior Change Strategies

■ Most of diabetes care is actually self-care that requires patients to actively participate in decision-making, goal-setting, and the process of daily management. Multiple behavioral changes are often required for patients to manage diabetes effectively and achieve their desired level of glycemic control.

■ Making and sustaining the behavioral changes needed for diabetes self-management requires collaboration between the patient and provider to develop a relevant useful plan.

■ To succeed, patients need diabetes education followed by ongoing self-management and psychosocial support. Involving the entire health care team in this process increases the likelihood of success.

Behavior Change Strategies

Diabetes requires considerable effort on the part of patients, regardless of the treatment approach. Patients are often asked to adjust eating patterns and selection of foods, increase their activity, monitor blood glucose levels, take multiple medications, lose weight, perform foot care, and make multiple decisions each day based on blood glucose levels, activity, and food choices. In addition to these behavioral changes, patients need to cope with the stresses and emotional impact of knowing they have a chronic illness that can result in multiple complications and premature death. While the use of more intensive regimens offers great hope for a healthier future, they also increase the complexity and demands for self-care and behavior change. Regardless of the type of treatment program, the patient is ultimately responsible for its implementation.

This responsibility for behavior change and self-care is based on three characteristics of diabetes: choices, control, and consequences. First, the choices that patients make each day in managing their diabetes have a greater impact on their outcomes than the decisions made by health care professionals. Second, patients are in control of their self-management behaviors. As health care professionals, we can educate, cajole, and attempt to motivate, but patients have control over the decisions they make once they return to their homes. They can also choose different recommendations to follow each day. Third, the consequences for these decisions accrue first and foremost to patients. Diabetes, including its daily management, belongs to the person with the illness.

INFLUENCES ON BEHAVIOR CHANGE

The level of behavior change required to manage diabetes is difficult for most people. In spite of the innate desire that most adults have to be healthy and live a long, independent life, it is often difficult to maintain the behaviors required for a lifetime of self-care. Whereas most patients want to reach the recommended levels of glycemic control, they also want diabetes to interfere as little as possible with their normal lifestyle and routines.

Diabetes self-management education is essential for behavior change. However, a one-time education program is generally not sufficient to sustain self-care behaviors over a lifetime of diabetes. Making and maintaining behavior changes requires considerable motivation on the part of most patients. While it is tempting to try to motivate patients through use of positive or negative reinforcement (e.g., praise, criticism, fear tactics), the type of motivation required to make and sustain behavior changes for chronic illness care is most effective when it comes from within the patient and is directed at changes that are personally valued and meaningful.

Research related to self-determination theory predicts that when patients are given autonomy (a sense of choices and self-initiation) and helped to identify what is important to them and to set goals, they are more internally motivated to care for their diabetes than when they are feeling controlled or pressured. In addition, feeling more confident about making and sustaining behavior changes (self-efficacy) and decisional balance (weighing positive and negative effects of behavior change) also influence behavior change. Cultural beliefs and values and family and other social support can also serve as positive or negative influences.

Psychosocial factors can also affect patients' abilities to make and sustain behavior changes. For example, depression is much more common among people with diabetes and can negatively affect self-efficacy and motivation. The majority of patients, including those with difficulty meeting glycemic goals, also indicate that diabetes causes emotional distress and that these concerns are rarely addressed in their interactions with health care professionals. Encouraging patients to talk about these feelings, and actively listening to their responses, is not only therapeutic but can help uncover issues that may be detrimental to the patients' self-management and quality of life.

For many years, behavior change was synonymous with patient compliance. Health care professionals were viewed as the authorities on diabetes care and patients were expected to adhere or follow their advice. However, patients often resisted professional advice as an encroachment on their autonomy. As a result, many patients jeopardized their physical health to maintain their sense of emotional well-being.

In contrast to this view are more patient-centered or collaborative models of diabetes care. Patients are increasingly recognized as the decision-makers and leaders in their own self-care. This approach is compatible with the Chronic Care Model for health care delivery, which is based on an active collaboration between patients and providers.

In this model, the role of health care professionals is to provide patients with knowledge and skills for informed decision-making; attempt to understand the patient's perspective about diabetes; acknowledge feelings, cultural, and family influences and values; and support patients' efforts in achieving self-selected diabetes care goals.

STRATEGIES FOR BEHAVIOR CHANGE

Strategies for behavior change are based on autonomy motivation and autonomy support. *Autonomy motivation* is the internal process that drives behavior change. Table 6.1 outlines questions to assess autonomy motivation.

Autonomy support refers to the behaviors that professionals explicitly use to enhance motivation and self-directed behavior change. One of the most powerful strategies that providers can use to provide this type of support is to assist in setting goals. Establishing collaborative goals with patients greatly increases the likelihood that patients will be able to achieve those goals.

Most patients will need assistance in learning to set meaningful, measurable, and realistic goals. Table 6.2 outlines a five-step process for goal-setting that supports collaboration. When setting goals, it is helpful to encourage patients to think of these as experiments rather than as absolutes that will result in a success or a failure.

Table 6.1 Assessing Autonomy Motivation

What about diabetes is causing you the most anxiety or distress?
What about this situation needs to change for you to feel better about it?
What will you gain if you make this change?
What will you have to give up?
How will you feel if things do not change?
On a scale of 1–10, how important is it for you to make a change in this situation?
What can you do to bring about this change?

Beginning the next visit by asking patients about their experiment and what they learned as a result sets the agenda for the rest of the visit and future goal-setting.

SELF-MANAGEMENT SUPPORT

Most studies indicate that sustaining behavioral changes is more difficult than making an initial change. The majority of patients will need ongoing follow-up and support to maintain the gains made through a self-management education program or initial goal-setting. This type of support includes following up on goals set; assisting with stress, distress, and coping; collaborating to solve problems and overcome barriers; providing information about new or different treatment options; and setting new goals or recommitting to or revising existing goals.

REDESIGNING PRACTICE TO SUPPORT BEHAVIOR CHANGE

Most health care delivery systems are designed to provide acute rather than chronic disease care. In recent years, there have been growing pressures on providers to see more and more patients in less time with fewer resources and support staff.

Table 6.2 Self-Directed Goal-Setting

Identify the problem
What is the most difficult or frustrating part of caring for your diabetes at this time?
Determine feelings and their influence on behavior
How do you feel about this issue? How are your feelings influencing your behavior?
Set a long-term goal
What do you want? What do you need to do? What problems to you expect to encounter? What support do you have to overcome these problems? Are you willing/able to take action to address this problem?
Make a plan for a behavioral step
What will you do this week to get started working toward your goal?
Assess how the experiment worked
How did it work? What did you learn? What might you do differently next time?

Table 6.3 Provider and Practice-Based Strategies to Support Behavior Change

Provider strategies

Stress the importance of the patient's role in daily self-care and decision-making to achieve outcomes.

Begin each visit with an assessment of the patients' progress toward goals, questions, and concerns.

Provide information about the costs and benefits of behavioral and therapeutic options.

Provide information about and referrals to diabetes self-management education programs, support groups, and community resources.

Close the loop at the end of each visit.

Practice-based strategies

Create a supportive patient-centered environment.

Use waiting time to provide information and behavioral support.

Supplement information provided to patients using technology.

Incorporate behavioral support into interventions coordinated by nurses, case managers, or other office staff members.

Replace individual visits with group or cluster visits.

Routinely refer patients to diabetes education and medical nutrition therapy.

Assist patients to select an area of behavior change that is supported by all staff members at each visit.

There are, however, strategies that providers can use to support behavior change among their patients with diabetes. Table 6.3 outlines health care professional and practice-based strategies that can support effective self-management. One strategy is to determine the patient's concerns at the start of the visit through use of a short form completed in the waiting room (see Table 6.4) or by simply asking the patient what issues he or she would like addressed during the visit. Another effective strategy is to "close the loop" at the end of the visit by asking patients to tell you what they understood, clarifying any misunderstandings, and then asking the patient to identify one behavior they will do to care for their diabetes before the next visit.

Not all self-management support needs to be done by physicians. Nurses or other trained office staff can meet with patients before the visit and assess progress toward goals, establish an agenda for the visit, and help set a new goal. Referral to other health care professionals outside the practice (certified diabetes educators, dietitians, case managers), education programs, support groups, lay health workers, and community resources can also provide this type of support.

SUMMARY

Behavior change is a critical aspect of diabetes care that greatly affects patients' outcomes and quality of life. Health care professionals have a significant role to play in supporting behavior changes made by patients to effectively manage their

Table 6.4 Diabetes Concerns Assessment Form

Please answer the following questions before your visit. Your answers will help ensure that your concerns are addressed.
1. What is hardest or causing you the most concern about caring for your diabetes at this time? (e.g., following a diet, medication, stress)
2. Please write down a few words about what you find difficult or frustrating about the concern you mentioned above.
3. How would you describe your thoughts or feelings about this issue? (e.g., confused, angry, curious, worried, frustrated, depressed, hopeful)
4. What would you like us to do during your visit to help address your concern? (Please circle the letters in front of all that apply.)
   A. Work with me to come up with a plan to address this issue.
   B. I don't expect a solution. I just want you to understand what it is like for me.
   C. Refer me to another health care professional or other community services.
5. I would like answers to the following questions at this visit:
6. I would like answers to these questions at some future visit:
7. Other (please explain)

Developed by R. M. Anderson and M. M. Funnell, Michigan Diabetes Research and Training Center, ©2005, The University of Michigan, http://www.med.umich.edu/mdrtc/profs/index.htm.

diabetes on a daily basis. They can provide information about diabetes and referrals for diabetes self-management education programs, stress the importance of the patients' role in their own outcomes, teach the skills involved in behavior change, set collaborative goals, and provide ongoing behavioral support to assist patients to make and sustain these critical changes.

BIBLIOGRAPHY

Anderson BJ, Rubin RR: *Practical Psychology for Diabetes Clinicians.* 2nd ed. Alexandria, VA, American Diabetes Association, 2002

Anderson RM, Funnell MM: *The Art of Empowerment: Stories and Strategies for Diabetes Educators.* 2nd ed. Alexandria, VA, American Diabetes Association, 2005

Bodenheimer T, Wagner EH, Grumbach K: Improving primary care for patients with chronic illness. *JAMA* 288:1775–1779, 2002

Funnell MM, Anderson RM: Changing healthcare systems and office practice to facilitate patient self-management. *Curr Diab Rep* 3:127–133, 2003

Funnell MM, Brown TL, Childs BP, Haas LB, Hosey GM, Jensen B, Maryniuk M, Peyrot, M, Piette, JD, Reader D, Siminerio LM, Weinger K, Weiss MA: National standards for diabetes self-management education. *Diabetes Care* 30:1630–1637, 2007

Glasgow RE, Davis CL, Funnell MM, Beck A: Implementing practical interventions to support chronic illness self-management. *Jt Comm J Qual Saf* 29:563–574, 2003

Skovlund SE, Peyrot M, on behalf of the DAWN International Advisory Panel: The Diabetes Attitudes, Wishes, and Needs (DAWN) program: a new approach to improving the outcomes of diabetes care. *Diabetes Spectrum* 18:136–143, 2005

Weiss MA, Funnell MM: *The Little Diabetes Book You Need to Read.* Philadelphia, PA, Running Press, 2007

Index

Other Titles From The American Diabetes Association

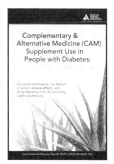
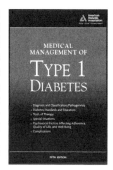
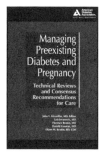
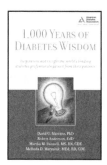